U0141395

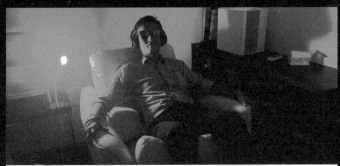

仲屏 **C.P** CHUNG PING 意識元宇宙

意識醫學 生物能 AI

Introduction the Technology of Consciousness Medicine

臨床教授：梁庭繼 醫師

從生物能的研究發展「意識醫學」
何謂「生物能」（BIOCERAMIC）？
「生物能」和最新量子物理學理論
「生物能」、「生物光能」、「生物能共振」和「生物能元宇宙」
生物能科技的國際性學術發表
生物能科技相關報導
生物能科技對睡眠品質、腦電波圖和腦部功能磁共振(fMRI)的影響
生物能科技在傳統醫學之應用
生物光能色彩醫學
生物能虛擬現實意識科技
生物能量意識—21「元宇宙」保健養生應用
生物能再生醫學
生物能星冠經絡數字
生物能智慧系統
執行中與進行中的意識醫學
十二銅人經絡代表穴位

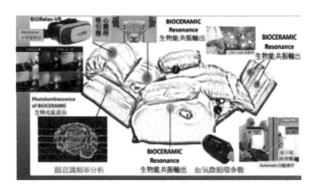

智能生物能系統概念

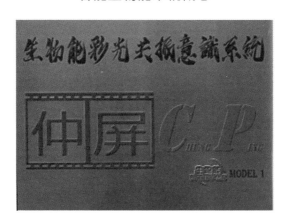

「仲」「屏」號 命名來自父母親---梁仲厚與梁錦屏名字

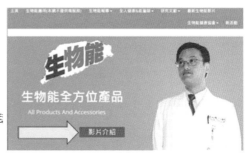

點選QR Code 可在生物能
資料庫連接教育影片
(youtube)

目　錄

序

「生物彩光共振意」識系統（元宇宙應用）讓您身心靈健康

　　臺北市生物能共振身心靈健康促進協會所倡導的
是：以科學的方法和理性的態度，透過生物能材料科
技，應用於生命和參透自然奧秘，可以加強描述 身(肉
體健康)、心(精神情緒健康)、靈(接觸五官五覺以外，
探索未知的宇宙空間) 進而促進身心靈健康，體驗天人
合一和發揮人道主義精神。

　　為什麼要倡導「身心靈」健康？而不是只倡導「身
體」健康呢？主要是一個『全人』的概念是，人除了有
形的「身體」之外，還有無形的「心靈」。現代西方醫
學主要是針對我們有形「身體」做疾病的治療與預防；
而「心靈」屬於無形、形而上的，在西方基督教稱為
「靈魂」，在東方道家稱為「元神」、較為科學的解釋
為「潛意識」的存在。

　　身心靈的能量彼此間常是互相牽引不止，互有影響
的。影響人類的能量，可以細分為『身心靈』三個部分
來看，亦即從身的能量、心的能量、靈的能量三方面來

4

探討。身心靈的能量彼此間常是互相牽引不止，互有影響的。本書是介紹『生物光能共振』技術如何幫助人們以『全人』保健醫學概念來協調維繫或重建『身心靈』或「身心意識」健康。

從生物能的研究發展「意識醫學」

摘要：

　　「意識醫學」是一種新興的跨學科範式，整合了物理科學、心理學、傳統醫學和意識研究元素，以提供一種全方位的健康方法。本綜述旨在闡明"意識醫學"的基本概念，重點探討生物能技術及其與人類意識和健康的互動。透過探索生物能技術、其對水性質的影響以及與傳統及替代療法的整合，本綜述全面概述了「意識醫學」如何將現代科學研究與整體療愈實踐相結合。

引言：

　　主流西方醫學一直專注於生物化學和分子生物學以應對健康問題。然而，主流醫學從未正式納入和承認一些生命的物理學現象，包括東方傳統醫學則關注非物質經絡通道的存在，包括西方傳統醫學所探討的反射區現象和影響情緒的物理「能量流」等客觀存在。另外，人類意識的複雜性及其對健康福祉的影響往往被忽視。

"意識醫學"是一個新穎的跨學科領域，旨在通過不僅整合生化和生理學見解，還理解意識和潛意識在健康和療愈中的角色來彌合這一差距。此方法考慮了生物能技術的深遠影響，通過一種弱生物力---「第五種基本物理力場」和光共振能量傳遞與生物系統甚至意識層次互動，從而影響身體、心理和感知狀態。

　　以下是根據我的有關我們四十多篇專門有關生物能研究的論文，基本架構出"意識醫學"的初步面貌，其開始於生物能的物理和化學研究（包括氫鍵），基礎醫學科學（體內和體外細胞和動物研究），人體研究，替代臨床醫學研究（包括傳統東方各傳統西方醫學），心理和精神科學研究，然後是意識（包括超感知覺）。最後的貢獻包括對人類「意識感知能力」水平的分類。

生物能技術與水的氫鍵結：

　　生物能技術能產生「第五種基本物理力場」，已被證明通過改變水的氫鍵結機制來影響其性質。水的基本性質，如黏度、表面張力和溶解度，受到氫鍵結動態性質的影響。研究表明，生物能技術會削弱這些鍵結，導致水的化學物理性質顯著變化。例如，處理過的生物能作用水表現出較低的黏度和表面張力，固體顆粒的溶解度增加，結晶溫度和酸度也發生了改變。這些變化顯示生物能技術通過其對水的影響可能調節細胞功能和整

體健康。

生物能技術的生物效應：

體外和體內研究：

體內外研究顯示，生物能技術能夠促進微循環，增強一氧化氮（NO）的合成，並調節鈣調蛋白（calmodulin），同時展現出抗氧化特性。例如，在成骨細胞和纖維母細胞中則增強了抗氧化活性。此外，在巨噬細胞和關節炎模型中，生物能技術能展現出抗炎效果，抑制前列腺素 E2、環氧合酶-2 和熱休克蛋白 70，同時優化水分子團，有助於調節炎症反應，維持組織健康，進而促進整體身體的健康和舒適感。這些生物效應與改善微循環和減少氧化應激密切相關，突顯了生物能技術在治療各種健康狀況中的角色。

中風康復和肌肉疲勞：

一系列已發表論文，針對缺血性中風模型的動物研究表明，生物光能技術通過改善微循環和周邊肌肉活動來增強運動功能和運動表現。這些模型中細胞內一氧化氮（NO）產生增加表明，生物能技術可能支持中風康復並減少肌肉疲勞，提供潛在的康復效益。

老鼠認知功能的影響：

老鼠老化通常由於氧化損傷和細胞功能失調而導致神經退行性症狀。有關生物能技術和彩色光研究顯示，這些干預措施可以改善老鼠的認知功能。該研究利用了不同波長的光和生物能，展示了在活動、認知和記憶方面的改善。值得注意的是，生物能技術與紅光結合在認知改善方面顯示出最顯著的效果，歸因於弱化的氫鍵結效應、改善的微循環和自主神經系統的增強調節。

而生物能技術與其中色彩藍光，綠光等結合，則有其他顯著改變。

生物能技術與東方傳統醫學---中醫的整合：

建立基礎醫學科學系統：

中醫藥長期依賴古籍和經驗知識，常常缺乏現代科學的驗證。生物能技術的整合為傳統與當代醫學實踐之間架起了一座橋樑。通過影響水性質和微循環，生物能技術符合中醫藥理論，並增強了對經絡和穴位的理解。這種整合支持更全面的方法來診斷和治療健康狀況，結合物質科學與傳統實踐。

經絡和穴位：

研究表明，經絡是非物質客觀存在，與心跳產生的一系列諧音頻率和駐波有關，在身體內形成特定的通道。生物能技術對微循環和生理狀態的影響支持這些中醫理論，這些理論認為經絡和穴位是能量流動的途徑。生物能技術可以通過優化經絡功能來增強內在能量平衡，進而促進身心健康的綜合效果。

生物能技術與西方傳統醫學的整合：

在名為《評估「生物陶瓷共振」操作下的反射區，透過受試者耳朵和的膀胱反射點進行同時刺激腳部，產生弱力場，導致受試者手部膀胱反射點電流變化》的美國替代醫學期刊的發表，我們通過這個實驗證明在生物能第五種力場的作用下，手掌、耳朵和腳底的反射區與人體特定內臟，是由一種看不見的信息鏈連接在一起，同時可以改善相關症狀。

意識醫學：整合治療的新典範：

意識醫學是一種整合身體、情緒和意識的全新健康照護方法，旨在促進整體健康。我們探討了意識研究在醫學領域中的發展，強調了基於證據的研究對於理解人體整體健康的重要性。特別引入了生物能共振技術，

作為一種潛在工具來探索意識的作用。進一步深入探討了利用生物能共振技術進行的試驗研究，以及其對意識狀態和超感知的影響。最後，討論了意識醫學在倫理、教育和未來發展方向上的重要性。

　　儘管現代醫學在治療身體疾病方面取得了顯著進展，但對於意識這一主觀存在的領域，我們的理解仍然有限。意識醫學因此應運而生，旨在填補這一知識不足。它提倡一種整全健康的模式，認識到身體、心靈和意識在促進健康中的密切聯繫。

　　在醫學史上，研究意識的探索具有深遠的根源。早期的學者們為我們理解心靈和身體之間的聯繫奠定了基礎。生物能技術的引入為我們提供了一種全新的途徑來研究意識及其對健康的影響。雖然這項技術的應用還需要進一步深入研究，但在探索意識狀態和其潛在療效方面已顯示出了角色定位。

　　意識醫學秉持整全健康的觀念，認識到身體、心靈和意識之間的緊密聯繫。一個領域的失調可能對其他領域產生深遠影響。通過整合傳統醫學實踐、心理治療以及增強靈性健康的技術，意識醫學致力於從綜合角度解決健康問題。

　　根據我們的研究結果，生物能刺激引發了多種不同等級的超感知現象和意識狀態改變，這些發現為我們深入了解生物能技術對人體的影響提供了重要的資訊。

在已經發表的研究論文，我們的研究檢視了 155 名受試者對生物能系統的主觀反應，以下是具體的描述：

約有 26.7% 的受試者為等級 0，表示未感受到任何明顯的改變或差異。這表明對生物能刺激的反應在某些人身上較低，或者反應不顯著。

約有 10.0% 的受試者在等級 1，表示感到放鬆，並在當晚獲得了更舒適的休息或睡眠。這顯示生物能可能對提升放鬆感和休息質量有所幫助。

約佔 48.7% 的受試者是等級 2，報告在皮膚上感受到不尋常的感覺，如增加的振動感、輕微的電感，以及在身體（尤其是經絡通道）中感受到的愉悅的輕鬆感。這些感覺可能反映了生物能刺激對身體能量流動的影響。

約有 8.7% 的受試者是等級 3，報告更深層次的感知，包括身體運動或旋轉感，以及視覺現象，如看到特定的顏色或光線。這表明生物能可能在促進身體能量流動和提升感知能力方面發揮了作用。

最後，約有 6.0% 的受試者是等級 4，報告了更複雜的聽覺和視覺現象，例如夢境般的幻象、離體經驗、透視或直覺的洞察力，以及與意識體的互動。這些深層次的體驗顯示了生物能刺激對意識的潛在影響，可能有助於深化對人體心靈互動的理解。

以上研究結果不僅豐富了我們對生物能技術的理解，還為進一步研究提供了堅實的基礎。通過深入探索不同等級的超感知和意識狀態改變，我們可以更好地理解生物能在促進整體健康和心靈發展方面的潛力。

　　根據我們的研究，57.1%的受試者選擇性超感知等級 4，其中大多數受訪者可視化不同形式的旋轉「曼陀羅」符號。這些符號源自印度哲學、佛教哲學、藏傳佛教徒、納瓦霍（美洲原住民）印第安人和基督教神秘主義者（如賓根的希爾德加德）中作為精神和儀式的象徵，代表宇宙的整體性和精神實體。此外，它們還出現在迷幻經驗中，尤其是使用 LSD、大麻、迷幻蘑菇、阿亞瓦斯卡等化合物時。從心理學家卡爾‧格的角度來看，這些視覺化可能反映了對整體性和秩序的心理追求，這些觀念在迷幻狀態和靈性體驗中尤為突出。

　　有了這些發現，我們進一步根據神經解剖學、生理學和醫學工程技術，開發針對松果體的能量刺激，以減少藥物和侵入性治療，幫助人們穩定情緒和精神狀態。我們發展了非侵入性的生物能技術，包括彩光能量和生物能共振，來刺激松果體。松果體本身是一個產生荷爾蒙的腺體結構，它利用常用胺基酸其一的色胺酸（Tryptophan）的化學結構轉化為血清素和退黑激素，甚至 DMT（N,N-二甲基色胺）。這些人體自行合成的

化學物質分別影響情緒狀態、晝夜節律、睡眠狀況和精神意識及幻覺的變化。

除此之外，根據過去的多項研究中証明侵入性傳統針灸手法在不同穴道的刺激，結合功能性腦部磁振造影（fMRI），證明了不同穴道針灸刺激會在腦部的不同區域產生功能變化。我們掌握了另一項技術，成功利用非侵入性的穿戴裝置來刺激經絡，從而觀察到腦部功能性磁振造影（fMRI）的變化以及量化型分頻率腦電波的頻率改變。這證實了非侵入性的生物能經絡刺激同樣可以改變人的意識狀態。

生物能元宇宙技術—針對身心症狀和情緒問題：

1.個體的情緒問題 醫學研究顯示，壓抑負面情緒或經歷挫折會顯著影響身心健康。基於「生物能光和聲音刺激-生物光子共振」技術的研究，臨床使用已顯示出顯著的改善情緒健康效果。利用腦功能磁振造影(fMRI)比較心因性睡眠障礙患者的治療前後結果發現，不僅症狀改善，還觀察到大腦和小腦相應區域的刺激現象，與精神疾病和情緒障礙有關。 近年來，抑鬱和不安情緒問題增加，尤其在青少年中影響巨大，造成家庭和學校的沉重負擔。有效篩查和及時干預可以避免不良後果，如過度依賴藥物、行為問題、自我傷害或自殺。

2.虛擬現實催眠（VR Hypnosis） 科學證據支持催

眠在疼痛管理中的有效性，且其使用得到臨床支持。然而，傳統催眠受限於治療師專業知識、時間和資源，使得提供催眠治療具局限性，且對患者來說，衡量催眠放鬆效果困難。 虛擬現實催眠（VR Hypnosis）通過三維、沉浸式虛擬現實技術引導患者進行放鬆、冥想、舒緩疼痛等，顯示出提高患者放鬆效果和治療效果的潛力。

3. 結合生物能---第五種基本力場導入身體後，利用現代元宇宙技術對意識進行引導，配合東方傳統和西方傳統保健醫學中的「內觀」、「動態圖像和符號」、「視覺與音樂或頻率」等刺激，產生超感知覺、情緒以及高層次意識的變化。

結論：

意識醫學代表著我們如何看待健康和福祉的重大轉變。通過將生物能技術與傳統醫學實踐、替代療法和心理研究相結合，這一領域提供了一個理解和增強人類健康的整體框架。探索生物能及其對水性質的影響，以及在意識醫學中的應用，強調了持續研究和跨學科合作的必要性。這種方法不僅擴展了我們對健康的理解，還提供了通過綜合和整合模型來改善福祉的創新途徑。

為了推進意識醫學的發展，需要進一步研究以驗證生物能技術在不同健康背景下的有效性。未來探索的

關鍵領域包括更大規模的臨床試驗、機制研究以了解潛在的過程，以及整合人工智能以優化治療方案。通過擴展對意識醫學的知識和應用，我們有望在革新醫療保健和促進更全面的健康方法方面取得成功。

總結：

　　「意識醫學」橋接了傳統與現代科學方法之間的差距，提供了健康的新視角。它整合了身體、心理和感知的多維度，補足過去主流西方醫學未重視的一些物理生命現象，包括東方傳統醫學所關注的非物質經絡通道的存在、西方傳統醫學所探討的反射區現象和影響情緒的物理能量流等客觀存在，以及人類意識的複雜性。通過對生物能及其相關技術的研究和應用，這一領域為更全面和包容性地理解人類健康和福祉打開了道路。

(一)何謂「生物能」(BIOCERAMIC)?

　　「生物能」有多種面相，包括「第五種力場」、「生物力場」和「超弱力場」。「生物能」是一種第五力場材料，是「電磁力場」、「引力場」、「強力場」和「弱力場」之外，人類發現的「新力場」，同時亦是一種「生物力場」和「超弱力場」。

　　在生物學中，「力場」的概念經過了一段很長，但一直受爭議的　史。要理解生命自然界有序的形式是怎

樣出現和運作，許多生物學家已經提出，除了生物化學過程和遺傳程式之外，有機體中必定有一種特殊的「生物力場」在其中作用。

　　早期的「生物力場」概念是由許多生物學家提出，其中包括前蘇聯的 N.K.科灰奔夫、匈牙利的 E. 鮑外和奧地利的 P.士斯。他們注意到了許多不能解釋的生物現象，例如海綿被分離的細胞能自發地重組起來，蠑螈殘留肢體(甚至眼睛虹膜)可以再生，以及有些物種的受精卵即使它們的亞分子結構被破壞，仍能夠發育成一個完整機體的能力。一種扁形虫被切成兩段時，它的「生物力場」會引導它重新長成一個完整的機體。有如一個被截成兩段的磁鐵形成兩個磁鐵，每個磁鐵都有它自己完整的磁場一樣。超越個人的交流活動特別經常出現在同卵雙胞胎之間。在許多情況下，一個雙胞胎能感覺到另一個所受到的疼痛，而且儘管其中一個遠在世界的另一邊，但另一個也能感知到他(或她)的傷痛和危難。除了"恋生疼痛"(twin pain)外，母親和子女間的敏感性也同樣值得注意。有數不清的事例表明，母親知道她的兒子或女兒在什麼時候遇到了大的危險或實際涉及到了某種事故。

　　有特別天賦的人能以「感覺」"進入"另一個人，尤其是如果他們是親戚或有深厚感情的話。感覺、聯想記憶和態度的轉移並不是唯一的一種超越個人的聯繫和交

流，這一點有明顯的證據。另一種則涉及意象的傳遞。除了思想轉移實驗外，塔格和普索夫逐進行過所謂的遙視" (remote – viewing) 實驗，在這些實驗中，發送者和接受者保持一定的距離，不可能有任何形式的 感覺交流。在隨機選定的一個地方，發送者作為一個"指路人"，然後接受者試圖看到指路人所看到的東西。傳統醫學現象中，異地身體效應是描述具有特殊能力的天生治病者產生的，這些天生的治病者"發送"他們稱 之為微妙的能量形式的東西到他們的病人那裡。科學家曾經檢驗發送者的心理意象對接受者的生理的影響。後者在很遠的地方感受到意象，但不知道這種意象是對著他們而來的。布勞德和施利茨聲稱已經證實:一個人的心理意象可以"越過"空間引起遠距離外的另一個人的生理變化。耶魯大學的生物學家 H.S.伯爾認為，「生物力場」是指引和組織生物體肉體結構的一種「生物力場」。伯爾的合作者 L.拉維茲聲稱他已經找到了「生物力場」在肉體死亡之前的一瞬間消失的證據。最近，像 B.古德溫生物學家証明，「生物力場」與植物和動物的生長過程有關。按照古德溫的觀點，當「生物力場」作用於現存的有機個體時，各種生命性質的形式就開始發展。「生物力場」是有機形式和組織的基本單位，分子和細胞僅僅是"合成的單位"。按照古德溫的觀點，生命的進化發生在有機體和環境的分界面上，再由

生物體和它們包含於其中的「力場」之間，相互作用所產生的神聖之舞的實現。古德溫不斷言「生物力場」獨立於生命有機體而存在，但是其他科學家，例如俄羅斯的生物學家 V.M. 伊紐欣，更直言不諱的說，「生物力場」是物理存在性的，無論它是否與生命有機體有關聯，這種「力場」是由離子、自由電子和自由質子組成的物質的「第五種狀態」。雖然對人類而言，這種力場附屬於大腦，也可以超越有機體表現出來，而產生心靈感應現象。英國植物生物學家 R.德雷克認為「生物力場」具有自身的實在性。謝爾德雷克看來，「生物力場」是一種"形態發生場"是由以前存在的同類有機體連續地塑造和加強所表現的，是物種的現有成員通過超越時空的因果聯繫與同物種的過去成員的形式聯繫在一起，這種聯繫通過「形態共振」方式發生，透過共振通過重復而得到加強，所以某一物種已經繁殖，它在未來就越是能繁殖，一種動物越是已經學會某種行為習慣，其他動物就能更快地學會這種行為習慣，如此等等。按照德雷克的觀點，「生物力場」---"形態發生場" 攜帶某種「不可測量的能量」。但是有關「生物力場」的証據卻另有說法。前蘇聯的波波夫生物資訊研究所的科學家們報告說，人類生物能量波長分散在 300-2000 毫微米(1 毫微米等於 100 位分之一米)的頻率範圍內變動。他們宣稱，這種「力場」與自然治療儀產生的效應有

關，治療儀的「力場」與病人的力場相互作用。蘭州大學的研究人員和上海原子核研究所的研究人員也已經開始研究人類「生物力場」的能量問題，他們發現這種「力場」隨著被試者的情緒和精神能力而變化。例如氣功師就比其他大多數人具有更高水準的「生物力場」。這一觀察已被洛杉磯加利福尼亞大學能量場實驗室的V.亨特的研究所証明。她利用由電路連接受試者和具有短程調頻數據傳輸的遙測裝置的精密儀器，通過把銀或氯化銀傳感器進到被試者身體的不同部位，測量人們的"情感改變部位"，她的測量顯示，受試者身體輻射能量的振動頻率會有所改變，同時觀察到「力場」強度與人類對顏色敏感度有相關性。亨特發現，以神秘主義者、預言家和特異功能治療者身上輻射出的能量場頻率測量範圍在 400 赫茲左右，遠比正常狀態下的人之能量場頻率測量範圍不到 250 赫茲高出很多。針對某些具有極高精神天資的個人所記錄下的"氣息場" (Aura)頻率往往高於 200 千赫茲，這是亨特儀器所能測量頻率的極限。因此，人類需要一個新理論，把「生物力場」對自然、生命和「身心靈」的解釋，重新建立在比過去所認知的，更微妙的時空相互關聯上。新紀元(New Age)學派科學家住住認為，宇宙萬物相互關聯是由全息(全像，holography)的信息編碼和傳輸的「超弱力場」所維繫的。一種具有全息(全像，holography) 維繫功能的「超

弱力場」在自然界中是存在的，物理學家以及生物學家已經發現了重要的証據，現在正等待這種革命性的發展，使人類在不斷探索真理的道路上有了下一個里程碑。(參考書: *The Whispering Pond*，*Ervin Laszlo*)

(二)「生物能」和最新量子物理學理論

要更了解「生物能」的作用和現象，必須先了解最新量子物理理論中的「超弦理論」(Superstring theory)和「M 理論」。

20 世紀初，物理學大師愛因斯坦突破了 19 世紀物理學瓶頸，分別以狹義和廣義相對論給人們一個新的物理圖像，其實對我們而言，愛因斯坦帶領人類認識，除了三度空間(維度)以外，原來還有第四度空間: (1 度空間=線<1D>、2 度空間=平面<2D>、3 度空間=立體<3D>和 4 度空間=立體+時間 <4D>)。

愛因斯坦是唯一能與牛頓相提並論的物理學家，一般人也許以為愛因斯坦最大的貢獻只有發現相對時間和質能等價 $(E_0 = mc^2)$ 理論。其實從物理的觀念來看，他最大的貢獻是發現彎曲四度空間時空的觀念來描述萬有引力現象(即建立在黎曼幾何上面的廣義相對論)，另外是光子的觀念和效應，就算是經過他的相對論提出一百年後的 2016 年初，人類才首次實驗証明了愛因斯坦年青時所提出的「引力波」存在的數學計算結果。但是，

愛因斯坦並沒有滿足于幾何學和力學的統一，他還進一步尋求把所有已知的物質粒子與所有已知的時空力結合在自身沒有「時同性」的統一理論矩陣中，愛因斯坦建立相對論之後自然地想到要建立一個「統一各力場的理論」或萬有理論(Theory of everything)，他花費了後半生近 40 年的主要精力但沒有成功。除了「引力場」和「電磁力場」之外，實際上自然界還存在另外兩種相互作用力－－「弱力場」和「強力場」。但是，一個讓「統一各力場的理論」或萬有理論(Theory of everything)無法成功建立的原因是:因為「引力場」實在太弱，在宇宙只有四個空間(維度)存在的假設下，無法進行統合運算。而到底「引力場」有多弱，它只有「電磁力場」的 100，000，000，000，000，000，000，000，000，000 分之一，所以，您可以用一塊磁鐵(電磁力場)來離空吸著一片鐵片，等於對抗了整個地球的地心引力(引力場)之總強度 。「引力場」難以理解的「弱」，導致了連愛因斯坦和他身故後的許許多多物理學家都沒有辦法解決如何統合四大力場的問題。另一方面，自然界中四種相互作用的主要「力場」中，除了「引力場」之外的三種「力場」，都可以利用量子理論來描述，「電磁力場」、「強力場」和「弱力場」相互作用力的形成是可以用假設相互交換 "量子" 來解釋的。但是，「引力場」的形成完全是另一回事，愛因斯

坦的廣義相對論是用物質影響空間的幾何性質來解釋「引力場」。在這一圖像中，瀰漫在空間中的物質使空間彎曲了，而彎曲的空間決定粒子的運動。量子物理學家也可以模仿解釋「電磁力場」的方法來解釋「引力場」，這時物質交換的"量子"稱為「引力子」，但量子化後的廣義相對論是不可重整的，因此，量子化的「引力子」和廣義相對論到目前都是相互不容的。在極端條件下，顯示了量子場論和廣義相對論自身的不完善。因此，要解決量子場論和廣義相對論相互不容的問題，人類針對量子場論和廣義相對論應該在一個更大的理論框架裡統一起來。現在這一更大的理論框架已初顯端倪，它就是「超弦理論」。簡單來說，「超弦理論」認為物質是由遠比「原子」和「夸克」更小，像"弦"狀的基本單元所構成，"弦"是很小很小的弦的閉合圈（稱為閉合弦或閉弦），閉弦的不同振動和運動就產生出各種不同已經知道的各種基本粒子。所以，我們所認知的物質實體，其實都只是由能量振動所組成的。偉大的二十世紀科學家 (包括發明交流電、電磁線圈(特斯拉線圈) ......等等的天才發明家)---- 尼古拉·特斯拉(Nikola Tesla)曾經說過：如果你想找到宇宙的秘密，請思考---能量，頻率和振動的形式 (*Nikola Tesla: "If you want to find the secrets of the universe, think in terms of energy, frequency and vibration."*) 。

「超弦理論」是人們拋棄了基本粒子是點粒子的假設，而真正的基本單元是一維弦的假設而建立的新理論，自然界中的各種不同粒子都是一維弦的不同振動模式。與以往量子場論和規範理論不同的是，超弦理論要求「引力場」的存在，也要求規範原理和超對稱。毫無疑問，將「引力場」和其他由規範場引起的相互作用力自然地統一起來是超弦理論最吸引人的特點之一。

　　後來，改進自「超弦理論」的「M 理論」出爐了，該理論認為，要完整描述宇宙需要「十一個」空間(維度)才夠解釋宇宙真相，而「引力場」可以同時存在所有的空間(維度)中，這就是前面所提到的，為什麼「引力場」相對很弱，而「引力場」不像其他三種力場可以順利用假設相互交換 "量子" 化來解釋 。所以，現在最被認為有機會可以完成「統一力場理論」，就是把所有的作用力都納入到同一個物理模型(調和量子理論和廣義相對論) ，就是納入到「超弦理論」和之後它的改良版本---「M 理論」架構中，希望成為「萬有理論」(Theory of everything)。在這裡，我們提出：「生物能」，一種有別於「電磁力場」、「引力場」、「強力場」和「弱力場」之外的「第五種力場」具有「生物力場」和「超弱力場」的特性的「力場」，如同「引力場」在「超弦理論」和「M 理論」的定義下，「生物能」力場亦同時存在於人類一般不容易感覺認知的四個

空間(維度)以外的其他空間(維度)中,而同時具有「第五種力場」、「生物力場」和「超弱力場」的特點。

(三)「生物能」、「生物光能」和「生物能共振」、「生物能元宇宙」

(a)我的研究團隊過去利用「第五種力場」---「生物能」材料做了廣泛的細胞實驗、動物實驗和人體實驗,已經驗證出本「生物能」的多項生物效應,包括細胞內一氧化氮和攜鈣蛋白的微量促進,「生物能」可刺激多種類細胞產生人體必需的微量物質、一氧化氮及攜鈣蛋白的缺乏,與許多現代人糖尿病、高血脂、動脈硬化、骨質疏鬆及高血壓等現代文明病,與我們健康生活息息相關,反之,許多學者提出,一氧化氮(Nitric Oxide)及攜鈣蛋白(Calmodulin)對於心臟的保養、糖類代謝、深度睡眠、學習能力及情緒行為有所輔助,最為名的例子是藥物「威而剛」,經由服用後,擴大了人體內一氧化氮的效能,由種種研究得知,「生物能」可以經由物理的作用,不需經由服用,即可對於人體的多個系統如循環系統、 呼吸系統、內分泌系統及神經細統等都提供絕佳的保健能量。明顯有效的抗氧化功能、幫助肌肉收縮、減少代謝酸的累積,可幫助肌肉運動後從疲勞回復的時間、動物和人體實驗結果得知有抗關節炎和減緩肌肉疼痛的效果。

(b)「生物光能」是利用光子能量把第五種力場材料「生物能」力場帶入遠處或進入人體。

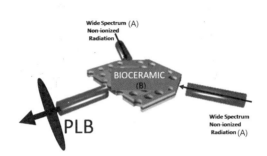

(c)「生物能共振」則利用特殊聲波能量把第五種力場材料「生物能」力場帶入遠處或進入人體產生駐波(standing wave)效應。

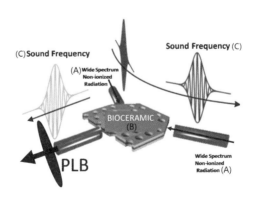

(d)「生物能元宇宙」是建築在「生物光能共振」第五力場所產生對人類意識提升現象的基礎上,而另外發展生物能虛擬實境平台……仲屏號意識系統。首先,要先解釋何為「意識」,一般來說,腦(brain)、意識(consciousness)、思想(mind)應該連在一起看。腦、意識是範圍比較小的層次,更高的層次是思想。在討論意識的時候,醫學界通常認為有兩種,一種是廣義的意識,包括自我意識,談的是主觀性的東西,它和精神醫學、心理學有關;另一種是狹義的意識,談的是客觀的東西,和腦神經生理學有關。「生物能元宇宙」—仲屏號意識系統,整合東方經絡、五行影音、道學內丹、 印度脈輪、正念冥想、神聖幾何動態曼陀羅、高頻波平衡頻率自然調理法(Rife/Spooky Frequency)等。

(四)生物能科技的國際性學術發表(40 篇)

Chinese Journal of Physiology 55(5): xxx-xxx, 2012
DOI: 10.4077/CJP.2012.BAA037

Effects of Far Infrared Rays Irradiated from Ceramic Material (BIOCERAMIC) on Psychological Stress-Conditioned Elevated Heart Rate, Blood Pressure, and Oxidative Stress-Suppressed Cardiac Contractility

Ting-Kai Leung[1, 2], Chien-Ho Chen,[3] Shih-Ying Tsai[4], George Hsiao[5], and Chi-Ming Lee[1, 2]

[1]Department of Diagnostic Radiology, Taipei Medical University Hospital
[2]Department of Radiology, School of Medicine, College of Medicine, Taipei Medical University
[3]Department of Laboratory Medicine, Taipei Medical University Hospital
[4]Department of Physiology, School of Medicine, College of Medicine, Taipei Medical University
and
[5]Graduate Institute of Pharmacology, Taipei Medical University, Taipei, Taiwan, Republic of China

Abstract

The present study examined the effects of BIOCERAMIC on psychological stress-conditioned elevated heart rate, blood pressure and oxidative stress-suppressed cardiac contractility using *in vivo* and *in vitro* animal models. We investigated the effects of BIOCERAMIC on the *in vivo* cardiovascular hemodynamic parameters of rats by monitoring their heart rates, systolic blood pressure, mean blood pressure and diastolic blood pressure. Thereafter, we assayed its effects on the heart rate in an isolated heart with and without adrenaline stimulation, and on cardiac contractility under oxidative stress

生物能之心血管保護

Property Characterization and Biological Function of High Far-Infrared-Emitting Ceramic Powders

林永昇、林明瑜、梁庭繼、廖啟宏、黃琼道、黃暉舜

Yung-Sheng Lin, Ming-Yu Lin, Ting-Kai Leung, Chi-Hung Liao, Tsung-Taio Huang, Hui-Shun Huang

遠紅外線是近年來熱門能事醫學領域之一。市場上述遠紅外線產品琳瑯滿目，但其遠紅外線輻射效事大都不高，生物效應垃垃有限。本研究開發了高效能遠紅外線陶瓷粉末，其成分為多種金屬氧化物之混合物，在生有光線 6－14 μm 之輻射高達 0.98 以上。實驗顯示此材料具有神菌效果，可細化水分子團而有助於細胞代謝，促進種子萌芽與生長，亦可提升茶葉之抗氧化能力。此外，對人體及皮體溫及微循環皆有提升之效果。由這些結果顯示，此遠紅外線材料日後將可廣泛應用於人類日常生活。

Far-infrared ray (FIR) is one of the topics in energy medicine which is hot for the past few years. There are numerous FIR products in markets but their FIR emissivities are almost insufficient and biological effects are quite limited. This study develops high efficient FIR-emitting ceramic powders composed of several metal oxides. The emissivity of this material in life light between 6 to 14 μm is above 0.98. Experiments reveal this material is antibacterial and it can miniature water clusters. The small water clusters can benefit cell metabolism, germination and growth of seeds and enhance in antioxidant activity of tea leaf. Besides it increase the skin temperature and microcirculation of human bodies. These results show this FIR material can be widely applied in human daily life in the future.

The applications of BIOCERAMIC technology on alternative therapy under the concept of traditional Chinese medicine

Ting-Kai Leung[1,2]

[1] Department of Radiology, Taipei Hospital, Ministry of Health and Welfare, Hsinchuang, New Taipei City, Taiwan

[2] Graduate Institute of Biomedical Materials and Tissue Engineering, College of Medical Engineering & Department of Radiology, Wan Fang Hospital, Taipei Medical University, Taipei, Taiwan.

Abstract

Photoluminescence of BIOCERAMIC and BIOCERAMIC resonance technology are based on applications of BIOCERAMIC material, which contains characteristics of non-ionizing radiation spectrum. In our past studies involved basic science, basic medical science and clinical science, we have already proved that it have weakening effect on hydrogen bonds of water and then enhance in vivo microcirculation, as well as other physiological functions. In this review article, we introduce its therapeutic effects, include: (i) model of diabetic animal on blood glucose control; (ii) model of stroke animal on improvement of post infarction exercise capacity; (iii) restore abnormal dermal surface mean current measurement of different acupuncture points; (iv) up regulate sensitivity

生物光能與生物能共振科技在臨床中國傳統醫學經絡應用

Contents lists available at ScienceDirect

Journal of Traditional and Complementary Medicine

journal homepage: http://www.elsevier.com/locate/jtcme

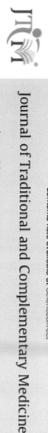

Establishment of a basic medical science system for Traditional Chinese medicine education: A suggestion based on the experience of BIOCERAMIC technology

Yuan Chia Chang [a], Ting Kai Leung [a, b, c, *]

[a] Department of Radiology, Taoyuan General Hospital, Ministry of Health and Welfare, No.1492, Zhongzhan Rd., Taoyuan Dist, Taoyuan City, 330, Taiwan
[b] Graduate Institute of Biomedical Materials and Tissue Engineering, College of Biomedical Engineering, Taipei Medical University, Taipei, Taiwan
[c] College of Health Care and Management, Kainan University, 33857 No.1 Kainan Rd. Luzhu, Taoyuan, Taiwan

ARTICLE INFO

Article history:
Received 18 August 2018
Received in revised form
16 April 2019
Accepted 21 April 2019
Available online xxx

Keywords:
BIOCERAMIC resonance
Meridians
Standing waves
Harmonic sound frequencies
Trigger points

ABSTRACT

The aim of this review study is to present an integrated and systematic approach to meridian channels and Ashi acupuncture points based on scientific evidence. We herein establish a framework of basic medical science to explain meridian channels based on the(1) Concepts of Traditional Chinese medicine(TCM) approach using physics and physiology: (i) the physical theory of pulse sound and cardio-vascular physiology: resonance of harmonic sounds and the specific frequencies arising from heartbeats, which form pathways of different meridian channels to enhance microcirculation; (ii) standing wave hypothesis to explain meridian channels; (iii) Ashi acupuncture or trigger points caused by ischemia due to inappropriate harmonic resonance of standing waves; and (2)the TCM concept strengthened by BIOCERAMIC technology: (i) 'wave-induced flow characteristics of meridians'; (ii) the Propagated sensation along meridian' phenomenon; (iii) clinical observations of the different chief complaints of candidates in which sensation was induced along specific meridian channels; (iv) generates 'biofield' phenomenon composed of virtual channels of interconnecting 'feet-hands-ears' to different internal organs/tissues that support the principles of reflexology.

生物能科技協助建立中醫基礎醫學教育

Biomedical Engineering: Applications, Basis and Communications, Vol. 32, No. 2 (2020) 2050021 (13 pages)
DOI: 10.4015/S1016237220500210

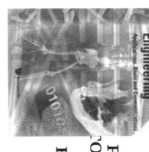

Biomedical Engineering
Applications, Basis and Communications

Original

EVALUATE CLINICAL EFFICACY OF BIOCERAMIC TECHNOLOGY ON PSYCHOPATHICALLY RELATED SPASMODIC TORTICOLLIS USING MOTION MEASUREMENTS, COMPUTERIZED ANALYSIS OF FACIAL EMOTIONS AND SPEECH SIGNAL FEATURES

Ting Kai Leung*,†,‡,||,**, Tzu-Sen Yang§,***, Ray F. Lin¶,**,

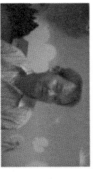

Frame 297

Frame 738

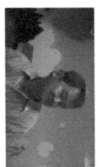

Frame 1146

Chula Med J Vol. 64 No. 3 July - September 2020;　　　　　　　DOI : 10.14456/clmj.2020.XX

Original article

Bioceramic resonance induced extrasensory perception or altered state of consciousness: A pilot study of Taiwan

Ting Kai Leung[a,b,c*]

[a]Department of Radiology, Taoyuan General Hospital, Ministry of Health and Welfare, No.1492, Zhongshan Rd., Taoyuan Dist., Taoyuan City 330, Taiwan
[b]Graduate Institute of Biomedical Materials and Tissue Engineering, College of Biomedical Engineering, Taipei Medical University, Taipei, Taiwan
[c]College of Health Care and Management, Kainan University, 33857 No.1 Kainan Rd. Luzhu, Taoyuan, Taiwan

Background: Our knowledge of consciousness is far behind other divisions of neuroscience.
Objective: Bioceramic resonance (BR) is a technology already applied to clinical medical services, it may help us gain knowledge on consciousness and cognitive neuroscience. This study is to evaluate the effect of BR on perception, state of consciousness and the related mental activity.
Methods: BR was applied on 155 adult subjects of Chinese who lived in Taiwan; they received questionnaire assessment of consciousness change or subjective response before and after using BR system. Further observations of selected cases for follow-up BR experiment. Precise descriptions and statistical analysis were performed on the results.
Results: Through the application of BR, participants (n = 155) reported specific perceptions, which include: (a) improvement in their sleep quality; (b) subjective sensation through certain parts of the skin; (c) deep swirling and light/color visualizations; and, (d) more intriguing cases involved candidates who had inexplicable phenomena with audio-visual experiences, such as rotating 'mandala'. In this study, we explain how BR affects different candidates with variable extrasensory perception experiences and alters the state of consciousness.
Conclusions: It is attempted to hypothesize that the BR effect may correlate with Jungian concept and the possibility of instrumentalization on psychotherapy. We conclude that BR is a non-invasive method, with potential benefits to neurological and psychological fields.

Keywords: Bioceramic resonance, extrasensory perception, consciousness, mandala.

Figure 3. She draw the image of 'mandala'(A) and a picture to record the three old men took a boat ride and the message telepathically input into her mind as '(written in Chinese) (B), that she visualized during the BR experiment.

Discussion

According to our result, as high as 57.1% of the selective extrasensory perception level 4 cases, had visualized different forms of rotating 'mandala' symbols. 'Mandala' is originated from Sanskrit, with the meaning an image of a 'circle' surrounded by a 'square'. It is usually act as a spiritual and ritual symbol in Hinduism and Buddhism, representing the universe.[9, 10] However, it also shared with Tibetan Buddhists, Navajo (Native American) Indians and

There are some limitations in this study. Experimental bias are not able to completely avoid, and the major limitations of this study are: (i) our results are based on subjective perceptions of different candidates; (ii) the lack of objective detecting device for data collection; and, (iii) the descriptions of their perceptions were not standardized, and were variables; this was as a result of their different education backgrounds.

生物能共振產生改變意識層次：台灣實驗初步成果

32

Leung T-K, et al., J Altern Complement Integr Med 2021, 7: 147

DOI: 10.24966/ACIM-7562/100147

HSOA Journal of Alternative, Complementary & Integrative Medicine

Research Article

Evidence-Based Approach and Discussion of 'Bioceramic Resonance' to Induce Altered States of Consciousness with Illusory Perception: Possible Application as a Complementary and Alternative Therapy

Ting-Kai Leung[1,2,3]* **and Yu-Ching Huang**[4]

[1]*Department of Radiology, Taoyuan General Hospital, Ministry of Health and Welfare, Taoyuan, Taiwan*

[2]*Graduate Institute of Biomedical Materials and Tissue Engineering, College of Biomedical Engineering, Taipei Medical University, Taipei, Taiwan*

with different categories of acute effect of stimulation, with different ratios from low to high levels of illusory perception based on their subjective descriptions and experiences induced by BR treatment.

Conclusion: By combing these results and our previous objective data of electroencephalographic brain wave activity and the locations of brain activation during 3T functional MRI scanning, we hypothesis that the phenomenon observed in this study mimics the psychotherapeutic effects of transcranial brain stimulation, which may probably explain by induction of cerebral electrical discharge and change of synchronous neuronal activity. We discussed the possibility of complementary and alternative therapy on different psychiatric and neurological disorders.

Keywords: Altered states of consciousness; Bioceramic Resonance; Cerebral electrical discharge; Illusory perception; Transcranial brain stimulation; Synchronous neuronal activity

Abbreviations

LTP: Left Temporal Pole
LPHG: Left Parahippocampal Gyrus

Review Article

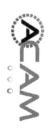

Complementary and Alternative Treatment of Using BIOCERAMIC related Technology on Mental and Psychiatric Related Disorders

Ting-Kai Leung[1,2,3*]

[1]Department of Radiology, Taoyuan General Hospital, Ministry of Health and Welfare, No.1492, Zhongshan Rd., Taoyuan Dist., Taoyuan City 330, Taiwan.

[2]Graduate Institute of Biomedical Materials and Tissue Engineering, College of Biomedical Engineering, Taipei Medical University, Taipei, Taiwan

[3]College of Health Care and Management, Kainan University, 33857 No.1 Kainan Rd. Luzhu, Taoyuan, Taiwan

Asian Journal of Complementary and Alternative Medicine. Volume 09 Issue 1

Published on: 25/02/2021

*Author for Correspondence: Ting-Kai Leung, Department of Radiology, Taoyuan General Hospital, Ministry of Health and

Digitalization and Tele-Health Care Concept of Complementary of Traditional Medical practices by Using BIOCERAMIC Technique

Authors: Leung, Ting Kai [1]; Tse Lin, Ming [2]; Lin, Shu-Chen [3];
Source: Acupuncture & Electro-Therapeutics Research
Publisher: Cognizant Communication Corporation
DOI: https://doi.org/10.3727/036012921X16304136917618

< previous   view fast track articles

... | ☰ | 99 | ☷
Abstract | References | Citations | Supplementary Data

Objective: Tele-health care service of alternative practice for chronic pain disease is worthwhile of developing, especially in the period of COVID-19 pandemic. Targeting on myofascial trigger points, this study was performed to assess the possible short-term pain relief and functional improvement in patients by applying the device of BIOCERAMIC material enhanced by frequencies of tempo sound and visible light spectrum (BioS&L).

Methods: Fourteen patients who participated in the procedure for the selection of trigger points for the BioS&L treatment, assessment of pain levels using a visual analog scale (VAS) analysis, and detection of abnormal resonance of 12 harmonic frequencies using a quantum resonance spectrometer (QRS).

Results: Comparing the pre-and post-treatment of BioS&L on pain score of 12 HFs(V1-V12) as measured by VAS estimated by mixed model showed 91.7% (11/12) improvement with statistically significant results. The distribution of differences in the QRS score estimated by the mixed model among participants with pre-test QRS level ≥ 2 showed 83.3% (15/16) of HFs with statistically significant results.

Conclusion: Treatment of BioS&L at trigger points providing pain relief is explained by the hypothesis of microvascular physiology and physics of wave propagation. This study provides a workshop with a concept of digitalization of complementarity and traditional medical service and tele-health care, which fulfils distant data connection and remote practice. In the period of epidemic spread, it helps to decrease close contact on both health care providers and patients.

Keywords: BIOCERAMIC; Rehabilitation; Trigger points; Visual Analogue Scale
Affiliations: 1: Radiology Dept., Taoyuan General Hospital, Ministry of Health and Welfare, No.1492, Zhongshan Rd., Taoyuan Dist., Taoyuan City 330, Taiwan. 2: Dept., Bioengineering, Taitung University, Taipei, Taiwan 3: Dept., Health Industry Management, Kainan University

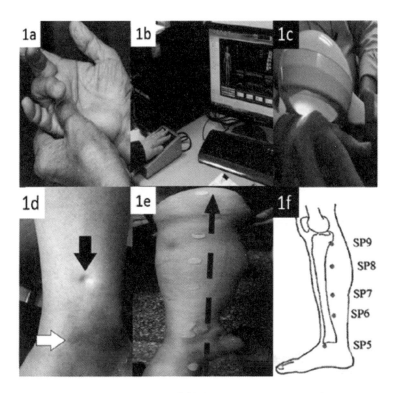

程醫療應用於傳統替代醫療服務的新概念

Journal of Medical and Biological Engineering, 33(2): 179-184

In Vitro Cell Study of Possible Anti-inflammatory and Pain Relief Mechanism of Far-infrared Ray-emitting Ceramic Material

Ting-Kai Leung[1,2,*]   Yu-Chuan Liu[2,3]   Chien-Ho Chen[4]   Hsieh Nien-Fang[1]

Kun-Cho Chen[1]   Chi-Ming Lee[1,2]

[1]Department of Diagnostic Radiology, Taipei Medical University Hospital, Taipei 110, Taiwan, ROC
[2]Faculty of Medicine, Taipei Medical University, Taipei 110, Taiwan, ROC
[3]Department of Biochemistry, Taipei Medical University, Taipei 110, Taiwan, ROC
[4]School of Medical Laboratory Science & Biotechnology, Taipei Medical University, Taipei 110, Taiwan, ROC

Received 26 Sep 2011; Accepted 26 Apr 2012; doi: 10.5405/jmbe.1029

Abstract

Inflammation and pain are the major chronic symptoms in geriatric medicine. This study examines the possible mechanism of a far-infrared ray-emitting ceramic material (bioceramic) on these symptoms using cell models. Effective doses of lipopolysaccharides (LPS) were added to induce acute episodes of inflammation in murine macrophage (RAW 264.7) and human chondrosarcoma (SW1353) cells. The inducible nitric oxide synthetase (iNOS), cyclo-oxygenase-2 (COX-2), and prostaglandin E2 (PGE2) levels were determined for the cell lines. Bioceramic treatment was found to have significant inhibitory effects on COX-2 and PGE2 and a probable effect on iNOS in the cell models of LPS-mediated inflammation. Bioceramic treatment may be an alternative method for palliative pain control to reduce chemical drug dependence for the protection of renal functions in the chronic pain disease population.

Keywords: Bone marrow stromal cells (BMSCs), Osteogenic differentiation, Collagen I nanospheres

醫用生物能消炎和止痛

37

Hindawi Publishing Corporation
International Journal of Photoenergy
Volume 2012, Article ID 646845, 8 pages
doi:10.1155/2012/646845

Research Article

Inhibitory Effects of Far-Infrared Irradiation Generated by Ceramic Material on Murine Melanoma Cell Growth

Ting-Kai Leung,[1] Chin-Feng Chan,[2] Ping-Shan Lai,[3] Chih-Hui Yang,[4] Chia-Yen Hsu,[3] and Yung-Sheng Lin[2]

[1] *Department of Radiology, School of Medicine, Taipei Medical University and Hospital, Taipei 110, Taiwan*
[2] *Department of Applied Cosmetology and Master Program of Cosmetic Science, Hungkuang University, Taichung 433, Taiwan*
[3] *Department of Chemistry, National Chung Hsing University, Taichung 402, Taiwan*
[4] *Department of Biological Science and Technology, I-Shou University, Kaohsiung 824, Taiwan*

Correspondence should be addressed to Yung-Sheng Lin, linys@sunrise.hk.edu.tw

Received 20 April 2011; Revised 9 July 2011; Accepted 9 July 2011

Academic Editor: Rodica-Mariana Ion

The biological effects of specific wavelengths, so-called "Far-infrared radiation" produced from ceramic material (cFIR), on whole organisms are not yet well understood. In this study, we investigated the biological effects of cFIR on murine melanoma cells (B16-F10) at body temperature. cFIR irradiation treatment for 48 h resulted in an 11.8% decrease in the proliferation of melanoma cells relative to the control. Meanwhile, incubation of cells with cFIR for 48 h significantly resulted in 56.9% and 15.7% decreases in the intracellular heat shock protein (HSP)70 and intracellular nitric oxide (iNO) contents, respectively. Furthermore, cFIR treatment induced 6.4% and 12.3% increases in intracellular reactive oxygen species stained by 5-(and 6)-carboxyl-2′,7′-dichlorodihydrofluorescein diacetate and dihydrorhodamine 123, respectively. Since malignant melanomas are known to have high HSP70 expression and iNO activity, the suppressive effects of cFIR on HSP70 and NO may warrant future interest in antitumor applications.

生物能體外抑制癌細胞

Direct and Indirect Effects of Ceramic Far Infrared Radiation on the Hydrogen Peroxide-scavenging Capacity and on Murine Macrophages under Oxidative Stress

Ting-Kai Leung[1],[*]   Yung-Sheng Lin[2],[3],[†]   Chi-Ming Lee[1]   Yen-Chou Chen[4]

Huey-Fang Shang[4]   Sheng-Yi Hsiao[3]   Hsuan-Tang Chang[1]   Jo-Shui Chao[1]

[1]Department of Radiology, Faculty of Medicine, Taipei Medical University and Hospital, Taipei 110, Taiwan, ROC
[2]Department of Applied Cosmetology and Graduate Institute of Cosmetic Science, Hung-kuang University, Taichung 433, Taiwan, ROC
[3]Instrument Technology Research Center, National Applied Research Laboratories, Hsinchu 300, Taiwan, ROC
[4]Graduate Institute of Medical Sciences, Taipei Medical University, Taipei 110, Taiwan, ROC

Received 16 Apr 2010; Accepted 17 Aug 2010; doi: 10.5405/jmbe 777

Abstract

Far infrared (FIR) rays are used for many therapeutic purposes, but the intracellular mechanisms of their beneficial effects have not been entirely elucidated. The purposes of this study were thus to explore the effects of ceramic-generated far infrared ray (cFIR) on RAW 264.7 cells by determining the scavenging activity of hydrogen peroxide (H_2O_2), cell viability, and changes in cytochrome c levels and the $NADP^+/NADPH$ ratios. The results showed that the H_2O_2-scavenging activity directly increased by 10.26% after FIR application. Additional FIR treatment resulted in increased viability of murine macrophages with different concentrations of H_2O_2. cFIR significantly inhibited intracellular peroxide levels and LPS-induced peroxide production by macrophages. The increased ratio of hypodiploid cells elicited by H_2O_2 was significantly reduced by cFIR. The effects of cFIR on H_2O_2 toxicity were determined by measuring intracellular changes in cytochrome c levels and the ratio of $NADP^+/NADPH$, and results showed that cFIR may block ROS-mediated cytotoxicity. In conclusion, data from this study suggest that cFIR may possess antiapoptotic effects by reducing ROS production by macrophages. We also review past articles related to the effects of oxidative stress from metabolically produced H_2O_2, and discuss possible beneficial effects of cFIR on living tissues.

生物能抗氧化強化免疫

39

Biomedical Engineering: Applications, Basis and Communications, Vol. 23, No. 2 (2011) 99–105
DOI: 10.4015/S1016237211002414

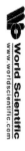

EFFECTS OF FAR INFRARED RAYS ON HYDROGEN PEROXIDE-SCAVENGING CAPACITY

Ting-Kai Leung[*], Huey-Fang Shang[†], Dai-Chian Chen[†], Jia-Yu Chen[‡],
Tsong-Min Chang§, Sheng-Yi Hsiao¶, Cheng-Kun Ho§ and Yung-Sheng Lin§,∥

*Department of Radiology, Faculty of Medicine
Taipei Medical University and Hospital, Taipei, Taiwan

†Department of Microbiology and Immunology, School of Medicine
Taipei Medical University, Taipei, Taiwan

‡Department of Dentistry, National Yang-Ming University
Taipei, Taiwan

§Department of Applied Cosmetology and Graduate Institute of Cosmetic Science
Hungkuang University, Taichung, Taiwan

¶Instrument Technology Research Center
National Applied Research Laboratories, Hsinchu, Taiwan

∥linys@sunrise.hk.edu.tw

Accepted 25 January 2011

ABSTRACT

Far infrared rays (FIRs) have several process effects on the human body and are generally considered to be biologically beneficial. In this study, we determined the effect of FIRs on hydrogen peroxide (H_2O_2)-scavenging activity, which was directly increased by 10.26% after FIR application. Even in the indirect use of FIRs accompanying carrot extract, FIRs still contributed to a 5.48% increase in H_2O_2-scavenging activity. We further proved that additional FIR treatment resulted in about 23.02% and 18.77% viability increases of antioxidant cells in the 300 and 800 μM H_2O_2, respectively, and about 25.67% and 47.16% viability increase of fibroblast cells in the 25 and 50 μM H_2O_2, respectively. Finally, FIR treatment also delayed senescence of detached *Railway Beggarticks* leaves in H_2O_2 solution with the concentration of 10, 100, and 1000 μM. By reviewing past articles related to the effects of oxidative stress from metabolically produced H_2O_2, we discuss possible benefits of FIRs for plants and animals.

生物能抗氧化強化生命力

Chinese Journal of Physiology 55(x): xxx-xxx, 2012
DOI: 10.4077/CJP.2012.AMM113

Bone and Joint Protection Ability of Ceramic Material with Biological Effects

Ting-Kai Leung[1, 2, *, #], Chien-Ho Chen[3], Chien-Hung Lai[4, 5, *], Chi-Ming Lee[1, 2], Chien-Chung Chen[6], Jen-Chang Yang[6], Kun-Cho Chen[1], and Jo-Shui Chao[1]

[1]Department of Diagnostic Radiology, School of Medicine, Taipei Medical University Hospital

[2]Department of Radiology, School of Medicine, College of Medicine, Taipei Medical University

[3]School of Medical Laboratory Science & Biotechnology, Taipei Medical University

[4]Department of Physical Medicine and Rehabilitation, School of Medicine, College of Medicine,

Taipei Medical University

[5]Department of Physical Medicine and Rehabilitation, Taipei Medical University Hospital

and

[6]Institute of Biomedical Materials Engineering, Taipei Medical University

Taipei, Taiwan, Republic of China

Abstract

Ceramic materials with biological effects (bioceramic) have been found to modulate various biological effects, especially those effects involved in antioxidant activity and hydrogen peroxide scavenging. As arthropathy and osteopathy are the major chronic diseases of geriatric medicine, we explored the possible activity of bioceramic on these conditions using animal and cell models. Rabbits received intra-articular injections of lipopolysaccharides (LPS) to induce inflammation that mimic rheumatic arthritis. FDG isotopes were then IV injected for PET scan examinations at 16 hours and 7 days after the LPS injection. We examined and compared the bioceramic and control groups to see if bioceramic was capable of relieving inflammation in the joints by subtracting the final and initial uptake amount of FDG (max SUV). We studied the effects in prostaglandin E2 (PGE2) inhibition on the human chondrosarcoma (SW1353) cell line, and the effects on the murine osteoblast (MC3T3-E1) cell line under oxidative stress. All the subtractions between final and initial uptakes of FDG in the left knee joints of the rabbits after LPS injection indicated larger decreases in the bioceramic group than in the control group. This anti-arthritic or inflammatory effect was also demonstrated by the PGE2 inhibition of the SW1353 cells. We further proved that bioceramic treatment of the MC3T3-E1 cells resulted in increased viability of osteoblast cells challenged with hydrogen peroxide toxicity, and increased alkaline phosphatase activity and the total protein production of MC3T3-E1 cells under oxidative stress. Since LPS-induced arthritis is an experimental model that mimics RA, the potential therapeutic effects of bioceramic on arthropathy merit discussion. Bioceramic may contribute to relieving inflammatory arthritis and maintaining bone health.

生物能促進骨骼與關節健康

41

Journal of Medical and Biological Engineering, 29(1): 15-18

Far Infrared Ray Irradiation Induces Intracellular Generation of Nitric Oxide in Breast Cancer Cells

Ting-Kai Leung[1,2]   Chi-Ming Lee[1]   Ming-Yu Lin[3]   Yuan-Soon Ho[2,4]

Ching-Shyang Chen[2,5]   Chih-Hsiung Wu[2,5]   Yung-Sheng Lin[3,*]

[1] Department of Radiology, School of Medicine, Taipei Medical University and Hospital, Taipei 110, Taiwan, ROC
[2] Breast Health Center, Taipei Medical University Hospital, Taipei 110, Taiwan, ROC
[3] Instrument Technology Research Center, National Applied Research Laboratories, Hsinchu 300, Taiwan, ROC
[4] Graduate Institute of Biomedical Technology, Taipei Medical University, Taipei 110, Taiwan, ROC
[5] Department of Surgery, School of Medicine, Taipei Medical University and Hospital, Taipei 110, Taiwan, ROC

Received 15 Sep 2008; Accepted 25 Nov 2008

Abstract

Far infrared (FIR) radiation has been used in many health-promoting applications, but the cellular mechanisms have not been elucidated. We investigated the influence of non-thermal-enhanced FIR for generating nitric oxide (NO) in breast cancer cells. We used MCF-7 breast cancer cells treated with FIR irradiation or left untreated, and measured

生物能促進一氧化氮

42

Biomedical Engineering: Applications, Basis and Communications, Vol. 21, No. 5 (2009) 317–323

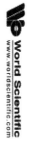

IMMUNOMODULATORY EFFECTS OF FAR-INFRARED RAY IRRADIATION VIA INCREASING CALMODULIN AND NITRIC OXIDE PRODUCTION IN RAW 264.7 MACROPHAGES

Ting-Kai Leung[*,†], Yung-Sheng Lin[‡,§,††], Yen-Chou Chen[¶],
Huey-Fang Shang[||], Yi-Hsuan Lee[**], Ching-Hua Su[||],
Huang-Chu Liao[*] and Tsong-Min Chang[‡]

[*]Department of Radiology, School of Medicine
Taipei Medical University and Hospital
Taipei, Taiwan

[†]Breast Health Center
Taipei Medical University Hospital
Taipei, Taiwan

[‡]Department of Applied Cosmetology and
Graduate Institute of Cosmetic Science
Hungkuang University, Taichung, Taiwan

[§]Instrument Technology Research Center
National Applied Research Laboratories
Hsinchu, Taiwan

[¶]Graduate Institute of Medical Sciences
Taipei Medical University, Taipei, Taiwan

[||]Department of Microbiology and Immunology
School of Medicine, Taipei Medical University
Taipei, Taiwan

[**]Department of Physiology, School of Medicine
Taipei Medical University, Taipei, Taiwan

生物能促進攜鈣蛋白

43

Original article

Textile Research Journal
82(11) 1121–1130
© The Author(s) 2012
Reprints and permissions:
sagepub.co.uk/journalsPermissions.nav
DOI: 10.1177/0040517512439917
trj.sagepub.com

Biological effects of melt spinning fabrics composed of 1% bioceramic material

Ting-Kai Leung[1], Jian-Miin Lin[2], Huan-Sheng Chilen[2] and Tzy-Chin Day[1]

Abstract

This study evaluated the usefulness of bioceramic materials (ceramic materials that emit high-performance far-infrared (FIR) rays), processed into fabrics using a traditional manufacturing melt spinning method. Numerous measurements were designed to test the biological functions of 1% bioceramic fabrics. These included physical induction of intracellular nitric oxide (NO) in NIH 3T3 cells (mouse fibroblasts), the effects on cell viability in osteoblastic cells (MC3T3-E1) under hydrogen peroxide-mediated oxidative stress, and the effects on lipopolysaccharide (LPS)-induced cyclo-oxygenase-2 (COX-2) and prostaglandin E2 (PGE2) production in a chondrosarcoma (SW1353) cell line. When compared to the control group, the bioceramic fabrics were capable of inducing further intracellular NO production using NIH 3T3 cells, and maintaining increased viability and against cell intoxication of osteoblastic cells by suppressing cell release of lactate dehydrogenase (LDH) under oxidative stress. In addition, it was found to suppress LPS-induced COX-2 production more significantly in a SW1353 cell line. These processes represent the biomolecular changes occurring during promotion of decline in aging, prevention of osteoporosis, and prevention of inflammatory processes within the human body. Therefore, these bioceramic fabrics are likely to fulfill their claims of having health-promoting benefits.

醫用生物能纖維

44

Hindawi Publishing Corporation
International Journal of Photoenergy
Volume 2012, Article ID 238468, 6 pages
doi:10.1155/2012/238468

Research Article

Inhibitory Effects of Far-Infrared Ray-Emitting Belts on Primary Dysmenorrhea

Ben-Yi Liau,[1] Ting-Kai Leung,[2] Ming-Chiu Ou,[3] Cheng-Kun Ho,[3] Aiga Yang,[3] and Yung-Sheng Lin[3]

[1] *Department of Biomedical Engineering, Hungkuang University, 34 Chung-Chie road, Shalu, Taichung 443, Taiwan*
[2] *Department of Diagnostic Radiology, Taipei Medical University Hospital & Department of Radiology, School of Medicine, College of Medicine, Taipei Medical University, 250 Wu-Hsing Street, Taipei 110, Taiwan*
[3] *Department of Applied Cosmetology and Master Program of Cosmetic Science, Hungkuang University, 34 Chung-Chie road, Shalu, Taichung 443, Taiwan*

Correspondence should be addressed to Yung-Sheng Lin, linys@sunrise.hk.edu.tw

Received 1 December 2011; Revised 21 May 2012; Accepted 5 June 2012

生物能抑制月經疼痛

Chinese Journal of Physiology 54(4): 247-254, 2011
DOI: 10.4077/CJP.2011.AMM044

247

A Pilot Study of Ceramic Powder Far-Infrared Ray Irradiation (cFIR) on Physiology: Observation of Cell Cultures and Amphibian Skeletal Muscle

Ting-Kai Leung[1, 2], Chi-Ming Lee[1, 2], Shih-Yin Tsai[3], Yi-Chien Chen[1], and Jo-Shui Chao[1]

[1]Department of Diagnostic Radiology, Taipei Medical University Hospital
[2]Department of Radiology, School of Medicine, College of Medicine, Taipei Medical University
and
[3]Department of Physiology, School of Medicine, College of Medicine, Taipei Medical University,
Taipei 11042, Taiwan, Republic of China

Abstract

The purpose of this research was to assess the potential for far-infrared ray irradiation from ceramic powder to improve exercise performance at room temperature. We designed experiments with murine myoblast cells (C2C12) to study the effect of cFIR irradiation on cell viability and lactate dehydrogenase release under H_2O_2-mediated oxidative stress and evaluated intracellular levels of nitric oxide and calmodulin. We also used electro-stimulation of amphibian skeletal muscle. Our results show that cFIR strengthened C2C12 under oxidative stress and delayed onset of fatigue induced by muscle contractions. We discuss possible mechanisms including anti-oxidation and prevention of acid build-up in muscle tissue based, and expect to see more applications of cFIR in the future.

生物能增強肌耐力

46

J. Chin. Chem. Soc., Vol. 58, No. 3, 2011

Physical-chemical Test Platform for Room Temperature, Far-infrared Ray Emitting Ceramic Materials (cFIR)

Ting-Kai Leung,[a,b]* Pai-Jung Huang,[c] Yi-Chien Chen[a] and Chi-Ming Lee[a,b]

[a] Department of Diagnostic Radiology, Taipei Medical University Hospital, Taipei, Taiwan, R.O.C.
[b] Department of Radiology, School of Medicine, College of Medicine, Taipei Medical University, Taipei, Taiwan, R.O.C.
[c] Department of Surgery, School of Medicine, College of Medicine, Taipei Medical University, Taipei, Taiwan, R.O.C.

Received December 17, 2010; Accepted March 3, 2011; Published Online March 17, 2011

Ceramic far-infrared (cFIR) emitting materials are sources of room temperature FIR radiation that allow non-thermal irradiation of biological tissue. In this study, we explored some interesting physical and chemical effects that have not been reported. We investigated the effects of cFIR irradiation of sorghum wine using gas chromatography with solid-phase micro-extraction (GC-SPME) to demonstrate enhancement on volatility; monitored pH changes resulting from irradiation on acetic acid; and used UV spectros-

生物能生產嚴謹---具科學驗證

47

CHINESE
CHEMICAL SOCIETY

DOI: 10.1002/jccs.201100491

The Physical, Chemical and Biological Effects by Room Temperature Ceramic Far-infrared Ray Emitting Material Irradiated Water: A Pilot Study

Ting-Kai Leung,[a,b,]* Jen-Chang Yang[c] and Yung-Sheng Lin[d]

[a] Department of Diagnostic Radiology, Taipei Medical University Hospital, Taipei, Taiwan, R.O.C.
[b] Department of Radiology, School of Medicine, College of Medicine, Taipei Medical University, Taipei, Taiwan, R.O.C.
[c] School of Dentistry, College of Oral Medicine, Taipei Medical University, Taipei, Taiwan, R.O.C.
[d] Department of Applied Cosmetology and Graduate Institute of Cosmetic Science, Hungkuang University, Taichung, Taiwan, R.O.C.

生物能水記憶現象

Far infrared ray (FIR) is non-ionizing electromagnetic radiation with wavelengths of 4-16 μm. Ceramic far infrared ray emitting materials (cFIR) are sources of FIR that exhibit only non-thermal effects at room temperature. Certain physical, chemical and biological effects of cFIR irradiation were investigated in this study that heretofore has not been well characterized. We demonstrated that cFIR irradiation reduced the size of water clusters, and significantly increased the freezing temperature of water. We also observed an

Evaluation of Reflexology by "BIOCERAMIC Resonance" Operation producing Weak Force Field during Simultaneous Acupoint Stimulation of Urinary Bladder Point on Subject's Ear Resulting in Electric Current Change on Urinary Bladder reflex Point on Subject's Hands, and Related New Research Finding

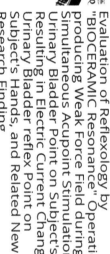

Abstract:

Objective: It was postulated in our previous publications that the meridian channels as conceived in Traditional Chinese Medicine (TCM) are various standing waves arising from harmonic rhythmic sound frequencies originating from the human heart beat. BIOCERAMIC is an artificial material able to produce a weak force field causing different biophysical and systemic health benefits, with the key characteristics of hydrogen bonds weakening and microcirculation enhancement. Since discovering that the effects of a BIOCERAMIC field can be transmitted via sound waves propagation, we then also developed a BIOCERAMIC Resonance device to produce weak force field throughout the body, and achieve resonance with the body's meridian channels to reinforce microcirculation. Methods: Since our previous research proved BIOCERAMIC can produces changes in ectodermal current levels, the present evaluation on reflexology is done by the application of Electric Current Detection (ECD) to the palmar surface of the hands matching correlative organs and glands loci to reflex points according to standard reflexology. The procedure will compare changes in the electrical current observed before and after a session of BIOCERAMIC Resonance treatment on the soles of the subjects' feet. We also conducted a procedure using corona discharge (Kirlian) photography of the hands to examine whether the coronal intensities could be affected by application of the BIOCERAMIC patch. Intensities are shown on the screen of a computer using special software that categorizes intensities into five zones. Results: Under the continuous treatment of BIOCERAMIC Resonance on soles of the feet and simultaneous stimulation on the specific zones of the ear representing the urinary bladder. The electrical current (Δµ ampere) on the areas in the hands are decreased from the beginning of the experiment, but only the specific area on the surface of the ear representing the urinary bladder was exhibited increased of the electrical current (Δµ ampere), with statistically significant difference (p<0.05). To the other study we evaluated the validity of reflexology and corona discharge (Kirlian) photography by applying BIOCERAMIC Resonance and small adhesive patches made from the BIOCERAMIC material. Significant differences were evident on four out of five different zones of the computerized images. Conclusion: Our findings suggest the existence of presupposed virtual channels or reflex points on the skin surface of the feet, hands, and ears that connect or somehow reflect back to specific internal organs, as mapped out on standard charts found in reflexology. Furthermore, the depicted corona intensities from five zones shown on a computer screen of the patches. This study demonstrates the operation of the BIOCERAMIC Resonance device is able to produce weak force field through the body, which is objectively measurable and thereby scientifically integrating the concepts of reflexology, meridian channels and biofield therapy.

生物能共振產生弱生物力場,同時驗證
和影響耳手足反射區和光場

49

Chinese Journal of Physiology 58(3): 147-155, 2015
DOI: 10.4077/CJP.2015.BAD294

Review Article

In Vitro and In Vivo Studies of the Biological Effects of Bioceramic (a Material of Emitting High Performance Far-Infrared Ray) Irradiation

Ting-Kai Leung

Diagnostic Radiology Department, Taipei Hospital, Ministry of Health and Welfare
Hsin Chuang District, New Taipei City 24213

and

Department of Diagnostic Radiology, Taipei Municipal Wanfang Hospital, Taipei City 11695,
Taiwan, R.O.C., Graduate Institue of Biomedical Materials and Tissue Engineering,
College of Oral Medicine, Taipei Medical University, Taipei 11031
Department of Radiology, School of Medicine, College of Medicine,
Taipei Medical University, Taipei 11031, Taiwan, Republic of China

Abstract

Bioceramic is a material that emits high performance far-infrared ray, and possess physical, chemical and biological characteristics on irradiation of water, particularly to in reducing the size of water clusters, weakening of the hydrogen bonds of water molecules and other effects on physical and chemical properties of water. In this review paper, we summarized the in vivo and in vitro biological effects of Bioceramic, and included previous published data on nitric oxide, calmodulin induction on cells, effects of Bioceramic on intracellular heat shock protein and intracellular nitric oxide contents of melanoma cells, antioxidant effects of Bioceramic on cells and plants under H_2O_2-mediated oxidative stress, effects on anti-oxidative stress of myoblast cells and on preventing fatigue of amphibian skeletal muscle during exercise, anti-inflammatory and pain relief mechanism, effects on the chondrosarcoma cell line with prostaglandin E2 production, effects on the rabbit with inflammatory arthritis by injection of lipopolysaccharides under monitoring by positron emission tomography scan, effects on psychological stress-conditioned elevated heart rate, blood pressure and oxidative stress-suppressed cardiac contractility, and protective effects of non-ionized radiation against oxidative stress on human breast

生物能於生物體內與試管之各項研究綜論

50

THE JOURNAL OF ALTERNATIVE AND COMPLEMENTARY MEDICINE
Volume 0, Number 0, 2013, pp. 1–7
© Mary Ann Liebert, Inc.
DOI: 10.1089/acm.2013.0122

Original Article

Effects of Far-Infrared Irradiation on Myofascial Neck Pain: A Randomized, Double-Blind, Placebo-Controlled Pilot Study

Chien-Hung Lai, MD, PhD,[1,2,*] Ting-Kai Leung, MD,[3,4,*] Chih-Wei Peng, PhD,[1,2] Kwang-Hwa Chang, MD,[1,5] Ming-Jun Lai, MD,[2] Wen-Fu Lai, DMD, DMSc,[6,7,8] and Shih-Ching Chen, MD, PhD[1,2]

Abstract

Objectives: The objective of this study was to determine the relative efficacy of irradiation using a device containing a far-infrared emitting ceramic powder (cFIR) for the management of chronic myofascial neck pain compared with a control treatment.

Design: This was a randomized, double-blind, placebo-controlled pilot study.

Participants: The study comprised 48 patients with chronic, myofascial neck pain.

Intervention: Patients were randomly assigned to the experimental group or the control (sham-treatment) group. The patients in the experimental group wore a cFIR neck device for 1 week, and the control group wore an inert neck device for 1 week.

Main outcome measurements: Quantitative measurements based on a visual analogue scale (VAS) scoring of pain, a sleep quality assessment, pressure-pain threshold (PPT) testing, muscle tone and compliance analysis, and skin temperature analysis were obtained.

Results: Both the experimental and control groups demonstrated significant improvement in pain scores. However, no statistically significant difference in the pain scores was observed between the experimental and control groups. Significant decreases in muscle stiffness in the upper regions of the trapezius muscles were reported in the experimental group after 1 week of treatment.

Conclusions: Short-term treatment using the cFIR neck device partly reduced muscle stiffness. Although the differences in the VAS and PPT scores for the experimental and control groups were not statistically significant, the improvement in muscle stiffness in the experimental group warrants further investigation of the long-term effects of cFIR treatment for pain management.

生物能於頸肌膜炎之臨床研究

51

Chinese Journal of Physiology 56(6): xxx-xxx, 2013
DOI: 10.4077/CJP.2013.BAB132

Physiological Effects of Bioceramic Material: Harvard Step, Resting Metabolic Rate and Treadmill Running Assessments

Ting-Kai Leung[1], Chia-Hua Kuo[2], Chi-Ming Lee[1], Nai-Wen Kan[3], and Chien-Wen Hou[2]

[1] Department of Diagnostic Radiology, Taipei Medical University Hospital & Department of Radiology, School of Medicine, College of Medicine, Taipei Medical University, Taipei
[2] Graduate Institute of Sports Sciences, Taipei Physical Education College, Taipei
and
[3] Center for Liberal Arts, Taipei Medical University, Taipei, and Graduate Institute of Athletics and Coaching Science, National Taiwan Sport University, Taoyuan, Taiwan, Republic of China

Abstract

Previous biomolecular and animal studies have shown that a room-temperature far-infrared-ray-emitting ceramic material (bioceramic) demonstrates physical-biological effects, including the normalization of psychologically induced stress-conditioned elevated heart rate in animals. In this clinical study, the Harvard step test, the resting metabolic rate (RMR) assessment and the treadmill running test were conducted to evaluate possible physiological effects of the bioceramic material in human patients. The analysis of heart rate variability (HRV) during the Harvard step test indicated that the bioceramic material significantly increased the high-frequency (HF) power spectrum. In addition, the results of RMR analysis suggest that the bioceramic material reduced oxygen consumption ($\dot{V}O_2$). Our results demonstrate that the bioceramic material has the tendency to stimulate parasympathetic responses, which may reduce resting energy expenditure and improve cardiorespiratory recovery following exercise.

生物能在耐久性運動時的節省能量與血氧消耗

52

Ting-Kai Leung Int. Journal of Engineering Research and Applications
ISSN : 2248-9622, Vol. 5, Issue 1(Part 2), January 2015, pp.85-94

RESEARCH ARTICLE

OPEN ACCESS

Photoluminescence of Bioceramic Materials and Bioceramic Resonance

Ting-Kai Leung[a],b

[a]Diagnostic Radiology department, Taipei Hospital, Ministry of Health and Welfare, Taiwan, China.
[b]Department of Diagnostic Radiology, Taipei Municipal Wanfang Hospital & Department of Radiology, School of Medicine, College of Medicine, Taipei Medical University, Taiwan, China

Abstract

The development of photoluminescent of BIOCERAMIC(PLB) and BIOCERAMIC resonance are based on BIOCERAMIC material, is a kind of non-ionized radiation spectrum emitting material possesses characteristics of weakening effect on water hydrogen bonds. The effect is corresponding to our previous medical-biological studies, such as microcirculation enhancement Herein, a review is to conclude our previous study on therapeutic effect of PLB or BIOCERAMIC resonance. They are include : glucose level control on diabetics by animal model; improved motor activity on middle cerebral arterial occlusion(MCAO) of rats by PLB treatment; normalizing ability to the mean current level measurement of acupuncture points on skin by PLB irradiation; enhanced propagated sensation along meridians; (PSM) phenomenon with clinical benefits by PLB effect on different meridian channels; combine effects of PLB and BIOCERAMIC resonance on many disorders such as insomnia, migraine(a chronic sympathetic nervous system disorder) and other autonomic nervous system disorder, associate clinical improvements; Thus, application of BIOCERAMIC technology for complementary therapy has scientific evidence based with good expectation.

Running title: BIOCERAMIC therapy

Key words: BIOCERAMIC; Resonance; photoluminescent; Meridian; Diabetics; parasympathetic; ANS

生物光能與生物能共振科技之應用

Lin et al., J Diabetes Metab 2013, 4:10
http://dx.doi.org/10.4172/2155-6156.1000321

Diabetes & Metabolism

Research Article

Photoluminescence of Bioceramic Materials (PLB) as a Complementary and Alternative Therapy for Diabetes

Shoei-Loong Lin[1,2], Cheuk-Sing Choy[3], Wing P Chan[4,5] and Ting-Kai Leung[5,6*]

[1]Department of Surgery, Taipei Hospital, Ministry of health and Welfare, Taiwan
[2]Department of Surgery, School of Medicine, College of Medicine, Taipei Medical University, Taiwan
[3]Emergency and Intensive Care Department, Taipei Hospital, Department of Health, Taiwan
[4]Department of Radiology, School of Medicine, College of Medicine, Taipei Medical University, Taiwan
[5]Department of Radiology, Wan Fang Hospital, Taipei Medical University, Taiwan
[6]Department of Physics, Fu Jen Catholic University, Hsinchuang, Taiwan
[7]Diagnostic Radiology Department, Taipei Hospital, Ministry of Health and Welfare, Taiwan

Abstract

The rapid rise of diabetes in Asia and Africa is surpassing that of western countries. Diabetes incurs a significant financial burden on patients and national economies. Consequently, factors such as a miserable life-long treatment of hypoglycemic therapy and the possibility of drug intolerance necessitate a search for non-pharmacological alternatives to reduce the requirement of anti-diabetic drugs. Photoluminescence refers to materials that absorb light energy and then release that energy in the form of light. In this study, Photoluminescence of Bioceramic Materials (PLB) was applied to control hyperglycemia and glycosuria in diabetes from the bench to the clinical bedside examination. The PLB treatments resulted in a tendency to promote glucose diffusion into C2C12 cell line and show a significant decrease in glycosuria in STZ (streptozotocin) induced diabetic rats. The possible mechanisms of the PLB effects on hyperglycemia also correlate with our previous publication and include molecular diffusion, calcium dependent nitric oxide, suppression of oxidative stress and autonomous nervous system regulation. In the future, PLB may have the role of clinical applications on ameliorating hyperglycemia and improving diabetes-related complications.

生物能生物光能改善高血糖

Translational Medicine

Research Article

Open Access

Lin et al., Transl Med 2013, 4:1
http://dx.doi.org/10.4172/2161-1025.1000122

Translating Laboratory Research of BIOCERAMIC Material, Application on Computer Mouse and Bracelet, to Ameliorate Computer Work-Related Musculoskeletal Disorders

Shoei Loong Lin[1], Wing Pong Chan[2], Cheuk-Sing Choy[3] and Ting-Kai Leung[2,4,*]

[1]Department of Surgery, Taipei Hospital, Ministry of health and Welfare, Taiwan, Republic of China

[2]Department of Diagnostic Radiology, Taipei Municipal Wanfang Hospital & Department of Radiology, School of Medicine, College of Medicine, Taipei Medical University, Taiwan, Republic of China

[3]Department of Emergency and intensive care, Taipei Hospital, Ministry of health and Welfare, Taiwan, Taiwan, Republic of China

[4]Department of Physics, College of Science and Engineering, Fu Jen Catholic University, Hsinchuang, Taiwan, Taiwan, Republic of China

[5]Department of Radiology, Taipei Hospital, Ministry of health and Welfare, Taiwan, Taiwan, Republic of China

Abstract

We investigated the effects of a room temperature-emitting far infrared ray ceramic material (BIOCERAMIC) on computer work-related pain and coldness. Thirty-two computer users reporting complaints in upper extremities and shoulders were assigned to play 30-cycles of specially-designed computer game. Each subject was provided with a normal and BIOCERAMIC-made mouse for the game on two different days. When using BIOCERAMIC mouse for the computer game, the most significant improvements among the upper extremity complaints were for wrist, finger, forearm, and partially shoulder soreness. Greater differences in surface temperatures of mouse and hand in BIOCERAMIC group were seen. The most significant difference occurred when using both the BIOCERAMIC cover and bracelet were found to reduce pain sensations. It was concluded that pain intensity and disability were significantly reduced after using BIOCERAMIC mouse for the game. The effect remained during follow-up when using BIOCERAMIC mouse cover and bracelet during their usual computer work.

生物能改善電腦工作相關肌肉骨骼疾病

55

Translational Medicine

Lin et al., Transl Med 2013, 3:1
http://dx.doi.org/10.4172/2161-1025.1000115

Enhancement of Transdermal Delivery of Indomethacin and Tamoxifen by Far-Infrared Ray-Emitting Ceramic Material (BIOCERAMIC): A Pilot Study

Shoei Loong Lin[1], Wing Pong Chan[2], Cheuk-Sing Choy[3] and Ting-Kai Leung[2,4,5*]

[1]Department of Surgery, Taipei Hospital, Ministry of Health and Welfare, Taiwan, Taiwan, Republic of China
[2]Department of Diagnostic Radiology, Taipei Municipal Wanfang Hospital & Department of Radiology, School of Medicine, College of Medicine, Taipei Medical University, Taiwan, Taiwan, Republic of China
[3]Department of Emergency and Intensive care, Taipei Hospital, Ministry of health and Welfare, Taiwan, Taiwan, Republic of China
[4]Department of Physics, College of Science and Engineering, Fu Jen Catholic University, Hsinchuang, Taiwan, Taiwan, Republic of China
[5]Department of Radiology, Taipei Hospital, Ministry of health and Welfare, Taiwan, Taiwan, Republic of China

Abstract

BIOCERAMIC have been found to modulate various biological effects. Our earlier published research on various cell lines demonstrated that BIOCERAMIC promoted microcirculation, upregulated calcium-dependent nitric oxide and calmodulin, and exerted an antioxidant effect by increasing hydrogen peroxide scavenging ability. The development of pain relief systems requires most possible minimum doses and methods for effective local control of pain, so as to protect liver and renal function. There is also clinical necessary to develop targeted delivery of estrogen inhibitor in the breast using a local drug release system, to protect the breast from the increased cancer risk associated with the use of estrogen therapy. We compared the viscosity of BIOCERAMIC irradiated water and control water, and found that BIOCERAMIC might weaken the hydrogen bonds. Such breaks are caused by the loss of hydrogen bond covalence resulting from electron rearrangement. The purposes of this study were thus to investigated a transdermal drug delivery model using Franz cell apparatus for indomethacin and Tamoxifen. The results showed that BIOCERAMIC might enhance the penetration performed by hydrogen bond weakening due to physical induction, and may facilitate local drug delivery in transdermal systems.

生物能促進經皮藥物吸收

56

Hydrology
Current Research

Leung et al., Hydrol Current Res 2014, 5:3
http://dx.doi.org/10.4172/2157-7587.1000174

The Influence of Ceramic Far-Infrared Ray (cFIR) Irradiation on Water Hydrogen Bonding and its Related Chemo-physical Properties

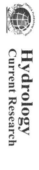

Leung TK[1,2,6], Lin SL[4], Yang TS[5], Yang JC[5] and Lin YS[6]

[1]Department of Physics, Fu Jen Catholic University, Hsinchuang, Taiwan
[2]Department of Diagnostic Radiology, Taipei Municipal Wanfang Hospital & Department of Radiology, School of Medicine, College of Medicine, Taipei Medical University, Taiwan
[3]Diagnostic Radiology department, Taipei Hospital, Ministry of Health and Welfare, Taiwan
[4]Department of Surgery, Taipei Hospital, Ministry of health and Welfare, No. 117, Su Yuan Road, Hsinzhuang, New Taipei City 242-13, Taiwan
[5]School of Dental Technology, Taipei Medical University, Taipei 110, Taiwan
[6]Department of Applied Cosmetology and Graduate Institute of Cosmetic Science, Hungkuang University, Taichung, Taiwan

Abstract

The property of water is highly related to the earth's environment and climate change. The fundamental dynamical process of water is include formation and breaking of hydrogen bonds. This dynamic process, so far, is still poorly understood. We investigated weakening of the hydrogen bonds of water after ceramic Far-infrared Ray (cFIR) irradiation and the resulting effects on physical and chemical properties of water. In this study, the Fourier transform infrared spectroscopy (FT-IR) was used to explore hydrogen bonding change of cFIR-irradiated water; in addition, capillary viscometers, Gas Chromatographs (GC), Differential Scanning Calorimetry (DSC), contact angles, Franz cells, High-Performance Liquid Chromatography (HPLC), and capillary electrophoresis analysis were used to evaluate its physical characteristics, such as viscosity, volatility, temperatures of water crystallization, surface tension, diffusion, hydrogen peroxide dissociation, solubility of solid particles, and changes in pH of acetic acid. The cFIR treated water decreased in viscosity and surface tension (contact angles), but increased in the solubility of solid particles, hydrogen peroxide dissociation, temperatures of water crystallization, and acidity of acetic acid. The weakening of water hydrogen bonds caused by cFIR irradiation is correspondent with our previous medical-biological studies on cFIR.

生物能弱化氫鍵，產生水質之物理化學變化

Journal of Medical and Biological Engineering, 34(1): 69-75

Protective Effect of Non-Ionizing Radiation from Ceramic Far Infrared (cFIR)-Emitting Material Against Oxidative Stress on Human Breast Epithelial Cells

Ting-Kai Leung[1,2,3*,†]   Chi-Ming Lee[1,4,†]   Shoei-Loong Lin[5]   Chih-Hsiung Wu[6,7]

Jeng-Fong Chiou[8]   Pai-Jung Huang[6]   Li-Kuo Shen[9,10]   Chin-Sheng Hung[1,6]

Yuan-Soon Ho[11]   Hung-Jung Wang[1]   Ching-Huei Kung[1]   Yi-Hsiang Lin[1]

Huey-Min Yeh[1]

[1] Faculty of Medicine, Taipei Medical University, Taipei 110, Taiwan, ROC
[2] Department of Diagnostic Radiology, Taipei Hospital, Ministry of health and Welfare, New Taipei City 242, Taiwan, R.O.C.
[3] Department of Diagnostic Radiology, Taipei Municipal Wanfang Hospital & Department of Radiology; School of Medicine, College of Medicine,
Taipei Medical University, Taipei 110, Taiwan, R.O.C.
[4] Department of Diagnostic Radiology, Cardinal Tien Hospital, New Taipei City 231, Taiwan, ROC
[5] Department of Surgery, Taipei Hospital, Ministry of health and Welfare, New Taipei City 242, Taiwan, ROC
[6] Department of Surgery, Taipei Medical University Hospital, Taipei 110, Taiwan, ROC
[7] Department of Surgery, Shuang Ho Hospital, Taipei Medical University, New Taipei City 235, Taiwan, ROC
[8] Department of Radiological Oncology, Taipei Medical University Hospital, Taipei 110, Taiwan, ROC
[9] Department of Radiology; Shuang Ho Hospital, Taipei Medical University, New Taipei City 235, Taiwan, ROC
[10] Department of Medical Imaging and Radiological Technology, Yuanpei University, Hsinchu 300, Taiwan, ROC
[11] Graduate Institue of Biomedical Technology, Taipei Medical University, Taipei 110, Taiwan, ROC

生物能降低輻射傷害、促進乳腺健康

58

Hindawi Publishing Corporation
Evidence-Based Complementary and Alternative Medicine
Volume 2016, Article ID 7230962, 9 pages
http://dx.doi.org/10.1155/2016/7230962

Research Article

The Effect of Photoluminescence of Bioceramic Irradiation on Middle Cerebral Arterial Occlusion in Rats

Lei Zhang,[1] Paul Chan,[2] Zhong-Min Liu,[3] Ling-Ling Hwang,[4] Kuo-Chi Lin,[5] Wing P. Chan,[6] Ting-Kai Leung,[6,7,8] and Cheuk Sing Choy[9]

[1] *Department of Radiology, Shanghai East Hospital, Tongji University, 1800 Yantai Road, Shanghai 200123, China*
[2] *Division of Cardiology, Department of Internal Medicine, Wan Fang Hospital, Taipei Medical University, No. 111, Sec. 3, Singlong Road, Taipei 116, Taiwan*
[3] *Department of Cardiac Surgery, Shanghai East Hospital, Tongji University, 1800 Yantai Road, Shanghai 200123, China*
[4] *Department of Physiology, Taipei Medical University, No. 250, Wu Hsing Street, Taipei 110, Taiwan*
[5] *Department of Diagnostic Radiology, Cathay General Hospital, 280 Renai Road, Sec. 4, Taipei 106, Taiwan*
[6] *Department of Radiology, Wan Fang Hospital, Taipei Medical University, No. 111, Sec. 3, Singlong Road, Taipei 116, Taiwan*
[7] *Graduate Institute of Biomedical Materials and Tissue Engineering, College of Medical Engineering, Taipei Medical University, No. 250, Wu Hsing Street, Taipei 110, Taiwan*
[8] *Department of Radiology, Taipei Hospital, Ministry of Health and Welfare, No. 127 Su Yuan Road, Hsinchuang District, New Taipei City 242-13, Taiwan*
[9] *Department of Emergency, Min-Sheng General Hospital, 168 Ching-Kuo Road, Taoyuan 330, Taiwan*

生物光能於腦缺血中風之應用研究

Hindawi Publishing Corporation
Evidence-Based Complementary and Alternative Medicine
Volume 2013, Article ID 739293, 11 pages
http://dx.doi.org/10.1155/2013/739293

Research Article

Wave-Induced Flow in Meridians Demonstrated Using Photoluminescent Bioceramic Material on Acupuncture Points

C. Will Chen,[1] Chen-Jei Tai,[2,3] Cheuk-Sing Choy,[4] Chau-Yun Hsu,[5] Shoei-Loong Lin,[6,7] Wing P. Chan,[8,9] Han-Sun Chiang,[10] Chang-An Chen, and Ting-Kai Leung[8,9,12,13]

[1] Department of Bioengineering, Tatung University, No. 40, Sec. 3, Zhongshan N. Road, Taipei 104, Taiwan
[2] Department of Traditional Chinese Medicine, Taipei Medical University Hospital, No. 252, Wu Hsing Street, Taipei 110, Taiwan
[3] Department of Medicine, Taipei Medical University, No. 250, Wu Hsing Street, Taipei 110-52, Taiwan
[4] Emergency and Intensive Care Department, Taipei Hospital, Department of Health, No. 127, Su Yuan Road, Hsinchuang, New Taipei City 242-13, Taiwan
[5] Graduate Institute of Communication Engineering, Tatung University, No. 40, Sec. 3, Zhongshan N. Road, Taipei 104, Taiwan
[6] Department of Surgery, Taipei Hospital, Ministry of Health and Welfare, No. 127, Su Yuan Road, Hsinchuang, New Taipei City 242-13, Taiwan
[7] Department of Surgery, School of Medicine, Taipei Medical University, No. 250, Wu Hsing Street, Taipei 110-52, Taiwan
[8] Department of Diagnostic Radiology, Taipei Municipal Wanfang Hospital, No. 111, Sec. 3, Hsing Long Road, Taipei 116, Taiwan
[9] Department of Radiology, School of Medicine, College of Medicine, Taipei Medical University, No. 250, Wu Hsing Street, Taipei 110-52, Taiwan

Hindawi

生物能光能無痛針灸效能研究

ACUPUNCTURE RESEARCH

Application of Photoluminescent Bioceramic Material for Different Chronic Illnesses by Selecting "Trigger Points" and "Propagated Sensation along Meridians" Phenomenon*

LEUNG Ting-Kai (梁廷繼)[1,2,3,4], Mimmo Gasbarri[5], TAI Chen-Jei (戴承杰)[6], and CHAN Wing P. (陳榮邦)[2,3]

· 1 ·

ABSTRACT Objective: To investigate the practicability on the processes of selecting "local tenderness skin points (trigger points)" and "propagated sensation along meridians" (PSM) phenomenon, and to find out the corresponding abnormal meridian channel in different illnesses. Methods: Ten patients with different kinds of chronic illnesses were administered photoluminescent bioceramic material (PLB) irradiations on meridians. The processes of selecting trigger points and PSM phenomenon were carried out on 80% (8/10) of the cases to find out the corresponding abnormal meridian channel in different illnesses. There were 8 cases identified by trigger points selection; 3 cases identified by PSM; 2 cases were not identified by either trigger points or PSM. These 2 cases were tested with electrodermal measurements of the 24 Ryodoraku meridian points to select their corresponding abnormal meridian channels for PLB irradiation. Objective and subjective Clinical improvements after PLB irradiations were recorded. Results: After PLB treatment, patients showed different noticeable improvements upon clinical observations. The most significant improvements were noticed shortly after subacute stage at 3–5 months durations of illnesses. Objective measurements showed a clinical improvement of 43.8%. Conclusions: To explain our clinical observations, we simply deduced that PLB treatment induced or promoted fluid/water diffusion along meridian channels. There was a gradually dredging of the meridian channels thus relieving stagnation and a vital change in the flow of dynamic patterns of the meridians. This conforms to, or validates, the old traditional Chinese theory of "Bu Tong Ze Tong" and "Tong Ze Bu Tong", that is, where there is obstruction, there is pain; where there is no obstruction, there is no pain.

KEYWORDS Chinese medicine, photoluminescent bioceramic material, Ryodoraku method

Found within the most important classical texts of Chinese medicine (CM) there is a particular axiom acupuncture points is a newly developed technique of which a series of scientific research was recently

生物光能經絡照射產生循經感傳現象，治療皮膚壓痛點

61

THE JOURNAL OF ALTERNATIVE AND COMPLEMENTARY MEDICINE
Volume 21, Number 8, 2015, pp. 472–479
© Mary Ann Liebert, Inc.
DOI: 10.1089/acm.2014.0076

The Analysis of Normalized Effects on Meridian Current Level After the Photoluminescent Bioceramic Treatment on Acupuncture Points

Ting-Kai Leung, MD,[1–4] Ming-Tse Lin, MSc,[5] Chang-An Chen, MSc,[6] Chau-Yun Hsu, PhD,[7] Shoei-Loong Lin, MD, PhD,[8,9] and C. Will Chen, PhD[5]

Abstract

Objective: This study investigated the advantage of photoluminescent bioceramic (PLB) irradiation on meridian channels of abnormal meridian currents, as well as the normalization of meridian current levels that may represent the participants' physiologic conditions.

Design: Statistical analysis of survey data.

Participants: Forty-six patients with abnormal meridian current in the gallbladder (GB).

Interventions: The effects on the meridian currents were measured by an electrodermal instrument after PLB irradiation was applied to the GB and other specific acupuncture points. Each meridian was categorized into six physiologic levels to evaluate effectiveness after the PLB irradiation: 1, extremely low; 2, moderately low; 3, normally low; 4, normally high; 5, moderately high; and 6, extremely high level. The positive effect of PLB treatment for each meridian could be defined as the normalized ability of the meridian level from the extreme values (1, 2, 5, or 6) approaching the normal levels (3 or 4).

Results: Participants with higher average meridian current (Amc >36 μA) calculated from the currents of 24 Ryodoraku points could be significantly normalized after the PLB treatment ($p = 0.0241$). A significant positive

研究合併生物光能與能量貼布應用
在恢復穴位點上經絡導電值的影響

Research Article

Bioceramic Resonance Effect on Meridian Channels: A Pilot Study

Ting-Kai Leung,[1,2,3,4] **Wing P. Chan,**[2] **Chen-Jei Tai,**[3,5] **Ting-Pin Cho,**[6] **Jen-Chang Yang,**[7] **and Po-Tsung Lee**[8]

[1] Department of Radiology, Taipei Hospital, Ministry of Health and Welfare, No. 127 Su Yuan Road, Hsinchuang, New Taipei City 242-13, Taiwan
[2] Department of Radiology, Wan Fang Hospital, Taipei Medical University, No. 111, Sec. 3, Xinglong Road, Taipei 116, Taiwan
[3] Graduate Institute of Biomedical Materials and Tissue Engineering, College of Oral Medicine, Taipei Medical University, No. 250, Wu-Hsing Street, Taipei 110, Taiwan
[4] Department of Radiology, Shanghai East Hospital, 1800 Yuntai Road, Pudong New Area, Shanghai 200123, China
[5] Department of Traditional Chinese Medicine, Taipei Medical University Hospital, No. 252, Wu Hsing Street, Taipei 110, Taiwan
[6] Metal Industries Research & Development Centre, 1001 Kaonan Highway, Kaohsiung 811, Taiwan
[7] School of Dentistry, College of Oral Medicine, Taipei Medical University, Taipei 110, Taiwan
[8] Department of Photonics and Institute of Electro-Optical Engineering, National Chiao Tung University, 1001 Ta Hsueh Road, Hsinchu 300, Taiwan

Correspondence should be addressed to Ting-Kai Leung; hk8648@tmu.edu.tw

Received 11 September 2014; Revised 16 February 2015; Accepted 16 February 2015

Academic Editor: Gerhard Litscher

生物能共振的醫學應用研究

Contents lists available at ScienceDirect

Journal of Traditional and Complementary Medicine

journal homepage: http://www.elsevier.com/locate/jtcme

Original Article

A technology developed from concept of acupuncture and meridian system, the clinical effect of BIOCERAMIC resonance on psychological related sleep disturbance with findings on questionnaire, EEG and fMRI

Lei Zhang [a, i], Paul Chan [b, i], Zhong Min Liu [c], Yi Li Tseng [d], C. Will Chen [e], Ming Tse Lin [e], Wing P. Chan [f], Ting-Kai Leung [g, h, *]

Under the concept of meridian channels that belongs to traditional Chinese medicine, BIOCERAMIC Resonance (BR) has already been applied to many clinical medical research projects with functions mimicking of traditional acupuncture. Forty-five patients were recruited with chronic sleep disorders; 36 patients were given, applied to the device with BIOCERAMIC material and sound rhythm on chest skin surface; 9 patients were included as controls. All study participants completed a sleep pattern and quality of life questionnaire (assessment on psychological and physical causes of sleep disturbances), which was repeated before, during and after treatment. Electroencephalograph (EEG) recordings were analyzed before, during and after treatment. Functional MRI (fMRI) was also used for demonstration of BR effect for another 8 candidates. During the first 3 days of treatment, sleep quality improved in all 36 patients especially to psychological reasons; in 91.7% (33/36) treatment was associated with an elevation in the beta spectrum of the EEG (at 15–27 Hz). The result of fMRI found corresponding cerebral and cerebellar areas of activation and deactivation. BIOCERAMIC Resonance can improve sleep disorder due to psychological causes, with transient alter brain wave activity and functional activation on specific locations of brain

生物能促進睡眠

Contents lists available at ScienceDirect

Journal of Traditional and Complementary Medicine

journal homepage: www.elsevier.com

ELSEVIER

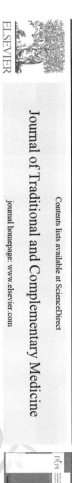

Base on concept of traditional Chinese medicine: Experimental studies on efficacy of BIOCERAMIC Resonance to alleviate drug withdrawal symptoms

Ting Kai Leung [*], Chi Ming Lee, Mimmo Gasbarri, Yung Che Chen

ARTICLE INFO

Article history:
Received 22 July 2017
Received in revised form 9 January 2018
Accepted 11 January 2018
Available online xxx

ABSTRACT

Those who are challenged by dependency on prescription drugs or suffer drug addictions have few options available to them for recovery, such as psychotherapy and physiotherapy. Here we present a new approach with clinical examples involving stimulant addiction or overdose of hypnotic drugs that were received BIO-CERAMIC Resonance, which was developed based on concept of 12 meridian channels of traditional Chinese medicine, and has successful withdrawal or dose reduction benefits. We describe the whole process and the clinical outcome. And by help of our previous publication on functional MRI, we discuss the possible brain lo-

生物光能共振戒毒/戒安眠藥之研究

65

healthcare

MDPI

Article

Disclosing Critical Voice Features for Discriminating between Depression and Insomnia—A Preliminary Study for Developing a Quantitative Method

Ray F. Lin [1,*] 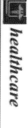, Ting-Kai Leung [2,3,†], Yung-Ping Liu [4] and Kai-Rong Hu [1]

† These authors contributed equally to this work.

Abstract: Background: Depression and insomnia are highly related—insomnia is a common symptom among depression patients, and insomnia can result in depression. Although depression patients and insomnia patients should be treated with different approaches, the lack of practical biological markers makes it difficult to discriminate between depression and insomnia effectively. **Purpose:** This study aimed to disclose critical vocal features for discriminating between depression and insomnia. **Methods:** Four groups of patients, comprising six severe-depression patients, four moderate-depression patients, ten insomnia patients, and four patients with chronic pain disorder (CPD) participated in this preliminary study, which aimed to record their speaking voices. An open-source software, openSMILE, was applied to extract 384 voice features. Analysis of variance was used to analyze the effects of the four patient statuses on these voice features. **Results:** statistical analyses showed significant relationships between patient status and voice features. Patients with severe depression, moderate depression, insomnia, and CPD reacted differently to certain voice features. Critical voice features were reported based on these statistical relationships. **Conclusions:** This preliminary study shows the potential in developing discriminating models of depression and insomnia using voice features. Future studies should recruit an adequate number of patients to confirm these voice features and increase the number of data for developing a quantitative method.

生物能針對情緒問題所衍生出之人功智能研究應用
成果

色彩生物光能改善學習與記憶能力，刊登於美國老化實驗研究期刊(SCI)

Experimental Aging Research ›
An International Journal Devoted to the Scientific Study of the Aging Process

Latest Articles

Submit an article   Journal homepage

Research Article

Effects of Bioceramic Material and Colored Light Irradiation on Learning and Memory in Aging Rats

Ting-Kai Leung, Yu-Chen Chen, Ming-Wei Chao & Chia-Yi Tseng

Received 29 May 2023, Accepted 27 Oct 2023, Published online 16 Nov 2023

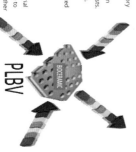

ABSTRACT

Aging is characterized by molecular damage from free radicals, leading to neural dysfunction and memory impairment. This study investigated using bioceramic material and colored light to mitigate neurodegenerative symptoms in aging rats. We assessed the effects of different color light spectrums on D-galactose-induced aging rats using the Morris water maze, novel object recognition, and open field tests. Findings revealed that bioceramic material with various light wavelengths improved activity, recognition, and memory in aging rats. Significant enhancements were observed in the open field and novel object recognition tests, with a trend toward improvement in the Morris water maze. These effects are attributed to the antioxidant properties and microcirculation enhancement associated with bioceramic materials. Color stimulation may impact enzymes, human physiology, psychological activity, and the autonomic nervous system. This study highlights the significance of exploring novel interventions for neurodegenerative symptoms and memory deficits in aging rats. Results indicate that bioceramic material with different colored light spectrums positively influences cognitive function. These findings contribute to our understanding of the therapeutic potential of bioceramic materials and emphasize the need for further research in this area.

（五）生物能科技相關報導

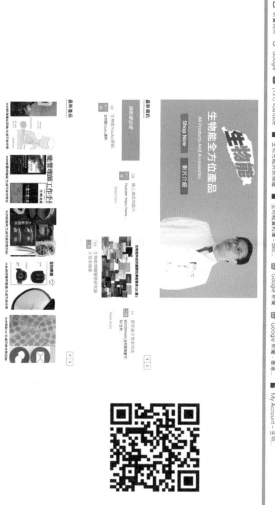

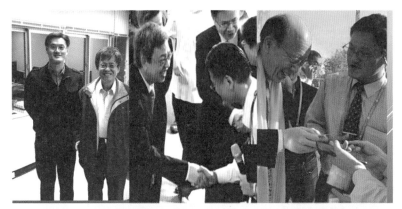

醫學能量的前輩:陳建德院士/陳建仁前副總統/李嗣涔前臺大校長

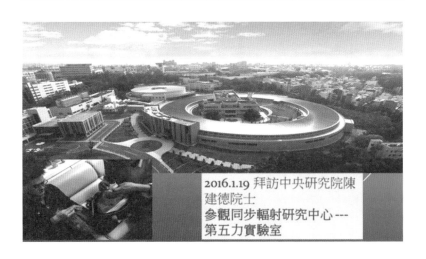

2016.1.19 拜訪中央研究院陳
建德院士
參觀同步輻射研究中心---
第五力實驗室

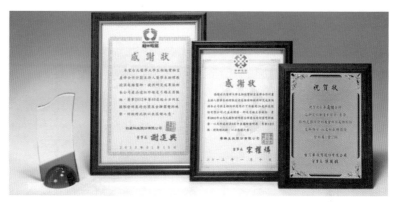

生物能實驗室
成果獲頒獎

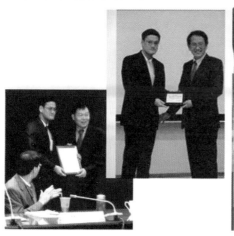

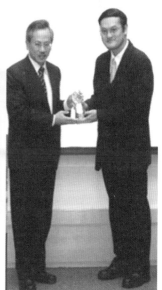

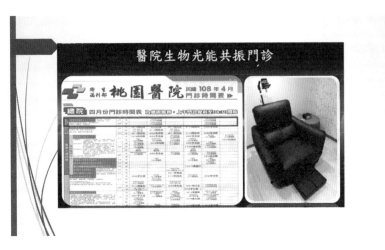

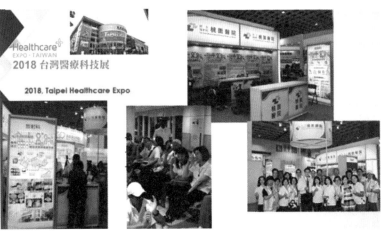

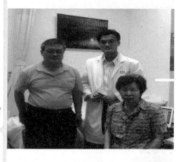

替代化學藥物治療的另類選擇
物理醫學--生物光能共振門診

光波和雷波共振所發生物理學材料，替代藥物效和失眠症、憂鬱症、病痛症...

生物光能共振是一種替代化學藥物治療的物理醫學，發展自振盪電磁輻射的生物陶瓷材料BIOCERAMIC (衛診醫製專章字第008331號)，所產生光波和雷波共振系統，發後伸至體內，應用傳統中國醫學，選擇不同頻率，與人體活官轉率共振，把生物能量帶進入體內來生和內部份官相調。創造出一些促進循環的良好環境，讓該患者化和身心疾病，所發的接受衣對替代醫學期刊 (Journal of Traditional and Complementary Medicine) 論文中，我們的生物能共振技術對身心症狀有改善效果，利用超聲波和31功能神經感測研發驗證本物的波生化和振盪和波震和的價值基礎。

「生物光能共振」針對失眠症、憂鬱症、病痛症等身心症狀有改善效果，可降低對化學藥品之依賴。另外，整合中醫與西醫的概念，以科學技術發展中醫經絡學說，針對慢性疼痛和關節疾病，包括婦女月經痛症、疲倦感、無法舉高的五十肩醫醫發現，有助養改善，可成為替代子宮和藥物治療的另類療症。

以科學論發現於2500年前成熟的「黃帝內經」所言：「通則不痛，不通則痛」，可以檢測為「共振自好會健康，共振不良會生病」，但作或出發表原者論文的國際學級醫學院刊第三十一篇，不斷更新並研和改良，「生物光能共振」技術存衛生署和桃園醫院門診服務病友。

台灣醫學大學醫師授

由於醫師群誠誠徵醫「生物光能共振」，門診全均異效

梁庭繼 醫師

學歷	台北醫學大學醫學士
經歷	高雄醫大附設醫院科學放射線主治醫師 ...

本院門診 乳房影像診斷（乳房攝影、乳房MRI、乳房intervention）... 一超醫學影像、介入性放射、醫學工程研究

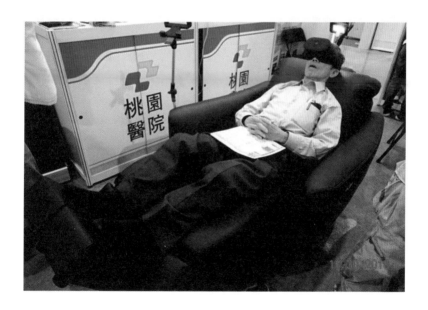

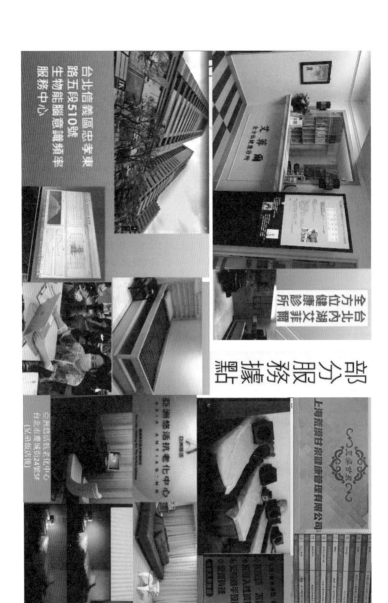

部分服務據點

全方位內湖健康艾菲診所爾

台北信義區忠孝東路五段510號
生物能腦意識頻率
服務中心

上海荒漠甘泉飛盟保健有限公司

亞洲樂活抗老化中心
ASIA ANTIAGING
台北市豫城街24號5F
（忠孝復興店後）

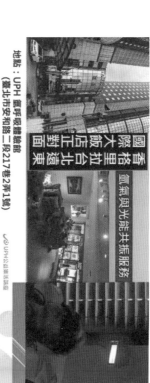

氫氧與光能共振服務

香格里拉台北遠東國際大飯店
（台北店正對面）

「生物光能共振」
抗氧化與強化傳統中醫的應用

UPH公益聯誼館

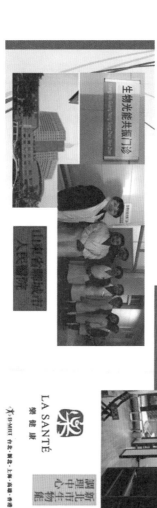

生物光能共振門診

山東省曹縣市人民醫院

地點：UPH 氫呼吸養鱗館
（臺北市安和路二段217巷2弄1號）

洽詢：(02) 2732-6131

報名：http://bit.ly/2PKBnZH

部分服務據點

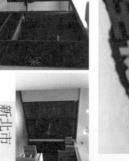

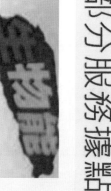

新北市中和自立路177巷2號店

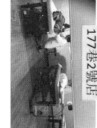

LA SANTÉ
樂健城

調理中市心生物能

新理北市心生物能

台北·新北·上海·高雄·神戶 B-MRT

74

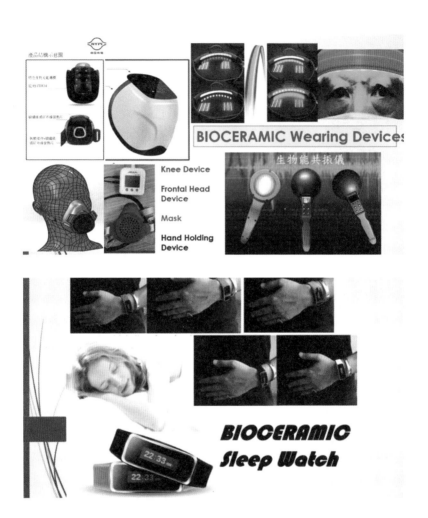

BIOCERAMIC Wearing Devices

Knee Device

Frontal Head Device

Mask

Hand Holding Device

生物能共振儀

BIOCERAMIC Sleep Watch

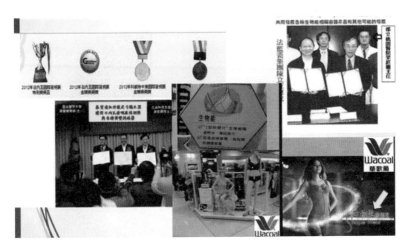

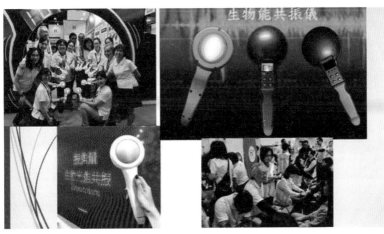

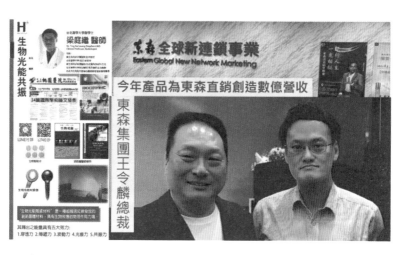

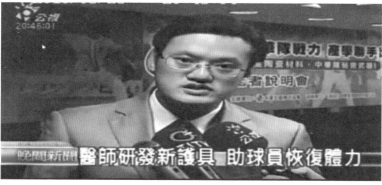

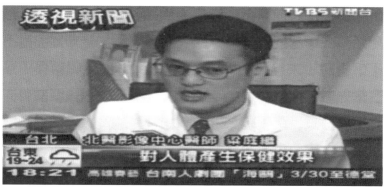

獨特優勢

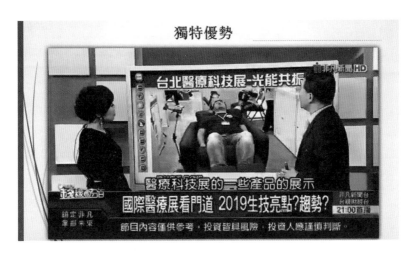

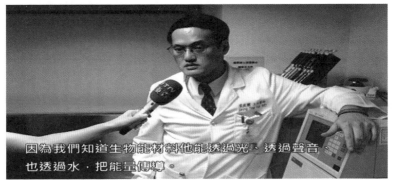

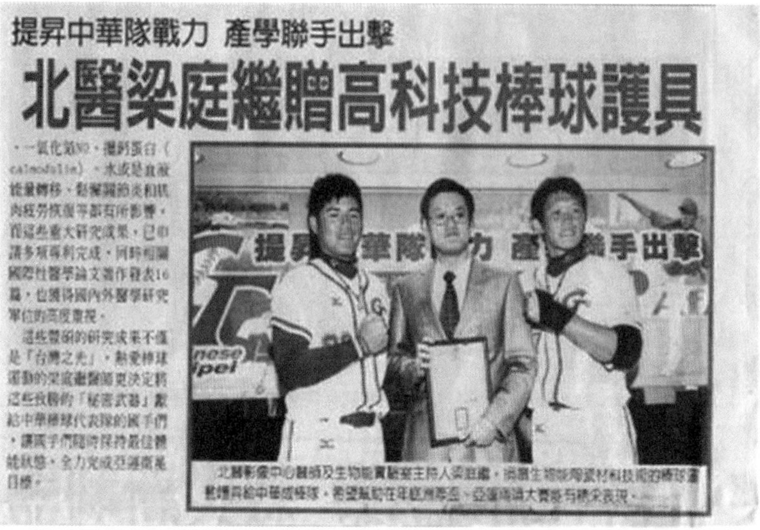

提昇中華隊戰力 產學聯手出擊

北醫梁庭繼贈高科技棒球護具

，一氧化氮NO、攜鈣蛋白（calmodulin），來改變自發能量轉移，對擊球的炎和抗肉疲勞恢復等都有所影響，而這些重大研究成果，已申請多項專利完成，同時相關國際性醫學論文著作發表16篇，也獲得國內外醫學研究單位的高度重視。

這些醫師的研究成果不僅是「台灣之光」，熱愛棒球運動的梁庭繼醫師更決定將這些致勝的「秘密武器」獻給中華棒球代表隊的國手們，讓國手們隨時保持最佳體能狀態，全力完成亞運爭冠目標。

北醫影像中心醫師及生物能實驗室主持人梁庭繼，捐贈生物陶瓷材料科技開發的棒球護具給中華成棒隊，希望幫助在年底[illegible]、亞運[illegible]大賽能有精采表現。

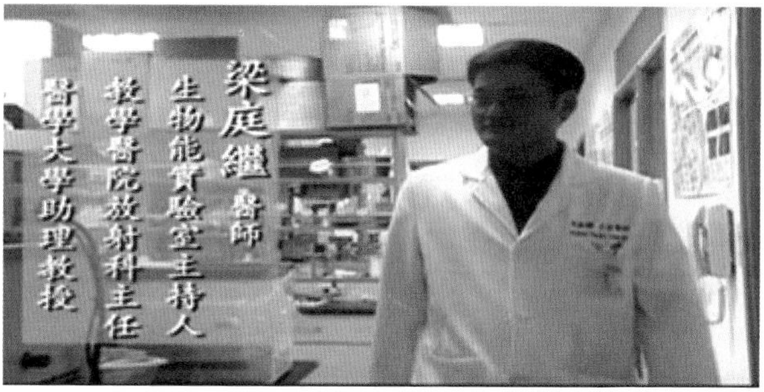
梁庭繼 醫師
生物能實驗室主持人
教學醫院放射科主任
醫學大學助理教授

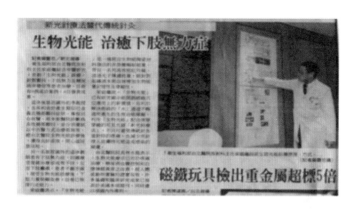

新光針療法代傳統針灸

生物光能 治癒下肢無力症

磁鐵玩具檢出重金屬超標5倍

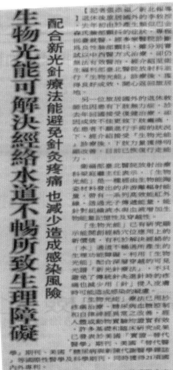

生物光能可解決經絡水道不暢所致生理障礙

配合新光針療法能避免針灸疼痛 也減少造成感染風險

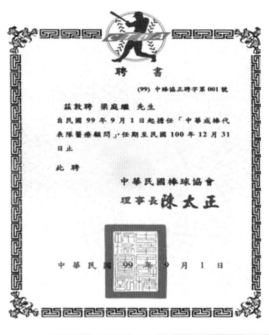

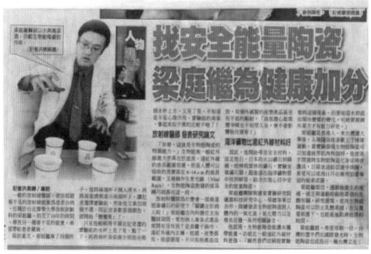

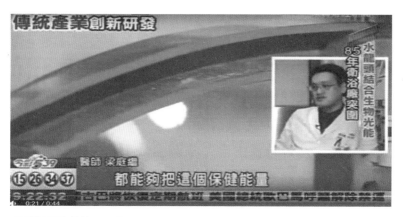

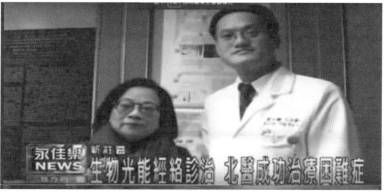

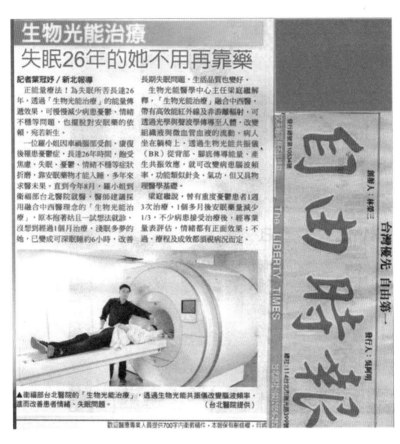

生物光能治療
失眠26年的她不用再靠藥

記者葉冠妤／新北報導

正能量療法！為失眠所苦長達26年，透過「生物光能治療」的能量傳遞效果，可慢慢減少病患憂鬱、情緒不穩等問題，也擺脫對安眠藥的依賴，宛若新生。

一位羅小姐因車禍腦部受創，康復後罹患憂鬱症，長達26年時間，飽受焦慮、失眠、憂鬱、情緒不穩等症狀折磨，靠安眠藥物才能入睡，多年來求醫未果。直到今年8月，羅小姐到衛福部台北醫院就醫，醫師建議採用融合中西醫理念的「生物光能治療」，原本抱著姑且一試想法就診，沒想到經過1個月治療，淺眠多夢的她，已變成可深眠睡約6小時，改善

長期失眠問題，生活品質也變好。

生物光能醫學中心主任梁庭繼解釋，「生物光能治療」融合中西醫，帶有高效能紅外線及非游離輻射，可透過光學與聲波學傳至人體，改變組織液與微血管血液的流動。病人坐在躺椅上，透過生物光能共振儀（BR）從背部、腳底傳導能量、產生共振效應，就可改變病患腦波頻率，功能類似針灸、氣功，但又具物理醫學基礎。

梁庭繼說，曾有重度憂鬱患者1週3次治療，1個多月後安眠藥量減少1/3，不少病患接受治療後，經專業量表評估，情緒都有正面效果；不過，療程及成效都須視病況而定。

▲衛福部台北醫院的「生物光能治療」，透過生物光能共振儀改變腦波頻率，進而改善患者情緒、失眠問題。　　　　（台北醫院提供）

相關報導

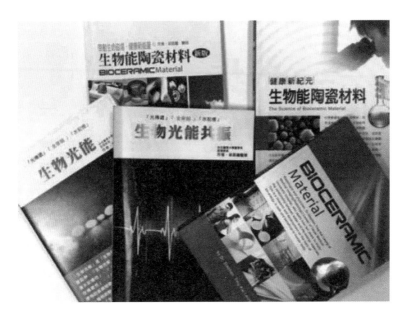

參考書籍

(六)生物能科技對睡眠品質、腦電波圖和腦部功能共振（fMRI）的影像

　　根據我們過去的臨床觀察，接受過生物能科技(包括:生物能、生物光能和生物能共振)的處置，往往發現睡眠障礙會得到改善，我們建立這項研究是通過對睡眠質量檢查和腦電波圖像的可能變化來更客觀評估生物能科技的有效性。

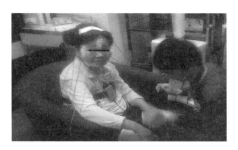
圖:腦電波實驗

　　透過「睡眠嚴重程度指數」和 「匹茲堡睡眠質量指數」的修改，我們使用了一種較適合台灣地區人民的自我評估問卷來進行數據收集，更能用於量化研究睡眠障礙的病人，同時協助進一步反映出心理性因素睡眠障礙或身體結構性因素睡眠障礙。比較接受生物能共振實驗人組（共 36 例）與未接受生物能共振(只有接受聲波拍子)對照人組（共 9 例）的結果，再進行統計分析。

　　本實驗為單盲測試實驗，受試者接受實驗時不知道被分配於生物能共振實驗組或是未接受生物能共振(只有接受聲波拍子)對照組。兩組都分別利用腦電波圖（EEG）數據記錄，均採用標準腦電圖頭皮線索和監督執行。受試者被告知實驗進行時不允許張開眼睛，記錄進行分析包括：生物能共振或未接受生物能共振(只有接受聲波拍子)作用前 15 分鐘，接受生物能共振或未接受生物能共振(只有接受聲波拍子)作用過程達 60 分鐘，和生物能共振或未接受生物能共振(只有接受聲波

拍子)作用後 15 分鐘。

圖：腦電波圖信號記錄（A1）:未接受生物能共振(只有接受
聲波拍子)作用前 15 分鐘，(A2):未接受生物能共振(只有
接受聲波拍子)作用過程達 60 分鐘，和(A3):未接受生物
能共振(只有接受聲波拍子)作用後 15 分鐘。

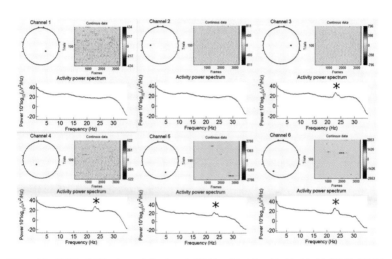

圖：前腦電波圖（EEG）信號記錄（B1）:生物能共振作用前
15 分鐘，(B2):在生物能共振作用過程達 60 分鐘，和(B3):
生物能共振作用後 15 分鐘。

作為未接受生物能共振(只有接受聲波拍子)作用的
對照組受試者，圖 A1-A3 中顯示出其中一個例子的結
果，但是包括作用前 15 分鐘，作用過程達 60 分鐘，和
作用後 15 分鐘，所述 EEG 信號沒有任何改變。相反

地，作為生物能共振作用的實驗組受試者，圖 B1-B3 中顯示出其中一個例子的結果，包括作用前 15 分鐘，作用過程達 60 分鐘，和作用後 15 分鐘，所述腦電波圖頻譜 15-27 赫茲範圍內明顯產生增生波，人數比例高達 91.7％（三十六分之三十三），同時具有統計學(使用 Fisher 精確檢驗統計比較)上的顯著增加 $P <0.05$）。

	對照組	實驗組
人數	9	36
腦電波圖頻譜 15-27 赫茲範圍內*沒有*產生增生波	100％	8.3％
腦電波圖頻譜 15-27 赫茲範圍內*明顯*產生增生波	0％	91.7％(P 值 <0.05)**

表: 統計學(通過使用 Fisher 精確檢驗統計比較)

(2) 睡眠情況問卷調查

Q1 不能在 30 分鐘內獲得睡覺
Q2 晚間醒來超過 30 分鐘以上
Q3 比預期醒來的時間提早 1～2 小時

Q4 來後沒有感覺神清氣爽
Q5 礙已經影響到白天的工作能力
Q6 疼痛或不適一直干擾睡眠
Q7 會因為情緒抑鬱或焦慮而干擾生活
Q8 因為打鼾引起呼吸暫停窒息
Q9 因有肢體和瘙癢等不適而防止入睡

實驗組和對照組都遵照指示於實驗完成三天後完成睡眠情況問卷調查。問卷包括九個問題（上表），統計分析(使用肯德爾秩相關係數，或 tau 蛋白試驗)進行比較實驗組（36 例）與對照（9 例），這是一種非參數假設檢驗以確定的睡眠障礙對治療反應的結果。

根據睡眠情況問卷調查評估結果，研究發現睡眠障礙改善為九個問題中的 Q1，Q2，Q3，Q4，Q5 和 Q7，都具有顯著性差異（P <0.05）;但不顯著性差異的是九個問題中的 Q6，Q8 和 Q9（P> 0.05）。

這些結果可能表明，問卷問題中的 Q1，Q2，Q3，Q4，Q5 和 Q7 因為比較反映由於心理因素產生的睡眠障礙，是較有可能透過生物能共振產生改善。然而，調查問卷中問題 Q 6，Q8 和 Q9 所反映的身體結構因素性睡眠障礙，則較未能透過生物能共振得到改善。

	tau-c	P 值
Q1	-0.210	0.003**
Q2	-0.170	0.016*
Q3	-0.169	0.016*
Q4	-0.165	0.022*
Q5	-0.191	0.004**
Q6	-0.105	0.139
Q7	-0.182	0.006**
Q8	-0.043	0.510
Q9	-0.084	0.222

表: 睡眠障礙情況問卷調查評估結果

結論

　　據我們所知，這是全球第一個臨床研究，以客觀數據證明一種物理方法可以改善心理因素產生的睡眠障礙和瞬間產生腦電波活動改變。我們認為，生物共振可以輔助或替代化學藥物(安眠藥)的使用。我們正使用功能性腦部磁振造影(fMRI)來進一步量化生物能對腦生理學的影響。

智能生物能科技協助減低安眠藥和精
神用藥，同時是傳統精神治療方式以
外的另一項選擇

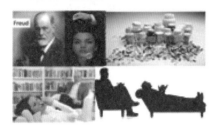

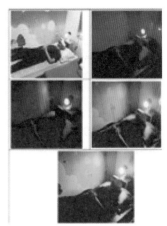

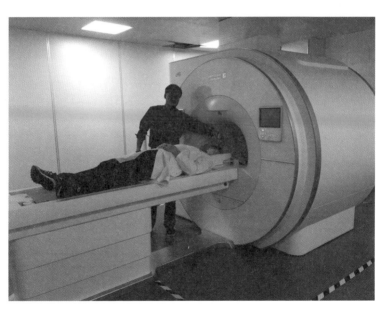

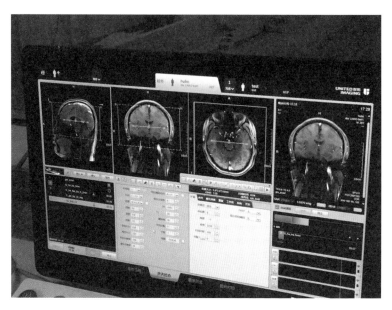

圖:功能性腦部磁振造影(fMRI)

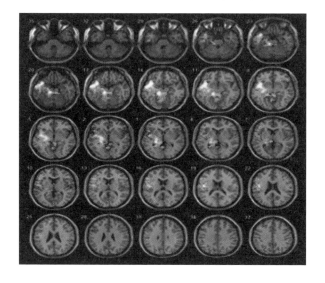

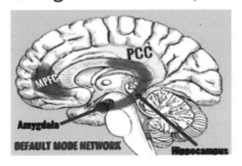

「預設模式網絡」
（DMN；default mode network）
「靜息狀態網絡」或稱（RSN；
resting-state network）

圖：「fMRI」腦功能性核磁共振---「預設模式網絡」（DMN
；default mode network）是研究人類潛意識存在的最新客
觀指標

（七）生物能科技在傳統醫學之應用

(1) 生物光能輸出：主要針對全身微血液循環，有
效改善失眠、偏頭痛、顏面神經顫抖症等自律神經系統
紊亂所引發的病症；改善糖尿病的血糖控制；改進中風
後的運動能力； 下肢腫痛(包括血管發炎)，另有淡化
皮膚黑色素等效果。請直接靠近患處使用照光，一次使
用時間十五分鐘以上，不限次數。

生物能共振輸出：輸出脈衝頻率之生物能波形，透
過可調控之生物能共振頻率來作用身體十二經絡，使

「生物能」量補充因心臟動脈共振和諧駐波共振不良的某特定十二經絡上。使用時身體儘量靠近把儀器輸出元件貼近皮膚，請先調至最高之生物能共振頻率，從低頻重高頻開始感受，如果身體某處慢慢有特別的痛或麻感(循經感傳現象)，代表這個生物能共振頻率(低頻或高頻)已有效產生該處所屬經絡之共振，同時代表該處所屬經絡共振不良，需要補充「生物能」量。但如果沒感覺，嘗試往低頻或高頻調動，有點像在使用傳統調頻收音機來找電台播放一樣。一般而言，有百分之 70 的人會感覺到身體某處慢慢有特別的痛或麻感(循經感傳現象)，但仍然有百分之 30 天生就不會感覺到，如果沒有找到，就調到最高頻率，繼續使用生物能共振，天生不會有循經感應傳導的人一樣會得到「生物能」好處。另外，如能配合使用「生物能」穴位貼，貼合在穴位和經絡線上(包括壓痛點和阿是穴)，會達到最好之效果。

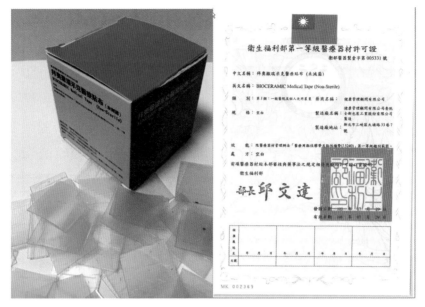

生物能穴位貼

中醫與西醫，以及東西方傳統醫學理論，應該可以整合一齊

首先我要介紹我的醫學教育與行醫背景，我因從小體質不好，28年前，在剛成為醫科學生的那些年，

參加了中醫社團，希望多明白一些養生知識，當時雖然能學習到許多針灸與中藥概念，可惜的事，與之同時，所接

受到的西醫課程，包括生理學、生化學、解剖學、藥理學和病理學等所集成之西方基礎醫學，發現中西兩者根本是無法相容，無從比較，兩者之學理更是無法相通。我

心裡相信中醫是有智慧和有價值的，但不能真正明白其原因。而天生具有好奇心、愛探索和追求真理，是我的本性，對此就一直感到失落。好不容易畢業後先從事內科住院醫師，我仍保有一股熱情，自資購買許多針灸材料，幫助我手上的病人和自我治療與保健；亦在業餘中，學習一些西方傳統醫學理論(包括：印度氣輪與歐洲同類療法等等)。

針對傳統醫學，我內心明確知有其真實性，卻不能為西方主流醫學和科學界所普遍認同。而一直以來，傳統醫學只能歸類在替代性療法(Alternative medicine)領域上。在台灣，雖然各大醫院都陸續開辦傳統醫學門診，但其實，各中西醫學家相互之間，難有高階學術互動，各自管理制度上，都不同。針對這一點，思考再三，本人提出以下看法：(1)傳統中西醫學的理論大部份是假設的，雖然擁有很複雜的學理與診療系統，卻沒有建立出以基礎科學驗證的事實，沒有建立客觀的基礎醫學；(2)與西方主流醫學相比較，各國沒有投入

足夠的人力物力來支援和幫忙傳統醫學進行最為基礎的科學研究，就無法使傳統醫學的科學理論建構起來，相關先進的傳統醫學專用診療儀器就無法研發出來；(3)傳統醫學缺乏如同西方主流醫學強大的知識系統，與臨床經驗的累積制度。就以中國傳統醫學家為例，因為各種可能原因，就算各中醫

師在其職業生涯中，經驗不斷累積，卻難有管道產生開方性的知識交流與經驗傳承，以致於各家各派各自運作；(4)由於傳統醫學家的臨床表現，除了要努力認真，對工作熱情外，其醫術精湛與否，很大是處決於其本人先天因素，是否擁有過人之大腦感受能力，來分辨病人身體上之輕細變化，例如傳統脈診的功夫，我個人認為，不是人人都有本事訓練出過人的觸感與把脈能力，當然就難以簡單傳承其醫術能力；(5)傳統醫學太注重古代經驗，大家讀的是古代文字，各人各自解釋其道理，缺乏統一思維，同時沒有現代精英編制出普遍可以遵循系統化的現代化文字綱要。

另一方面，基於我本身對研究的興趣，接下來我轉行為放射科專科醫師，同時在大學成立自己實驗室，誇領域從事非游離輻射的生物能量材料研發，進而進行其基礎醫學和臨床應用研究。諷刺的是，明明知道經絡穴位與氣輪的真實性，從事

多年的影像醫學工作(包括判圖 CT、MRI 與 PET 等)，卻從來無法以所學的醫學影像工作中看到過它們的存在。不過，應該是上帝的指引，擁有極度好奇的本性，我在「生物能量材料」(BIOCERAMIC)的研究成果和基礎上，另外開發了「生物光能治療儀」與「生物能共振治療儀」，開始利用自己發明的儀器，針對傳統中國醫學所提到的單穴位、單經絡、和不同穴位點與經絡所屬皮膚位置

的導電性、相互連動性，以及臨床上「循經感傳」(propagated sensation along Meridians)的真實性，作出研究；另外針對儀器在多種慢性疾病的療效分析。很快就有了客觀性結論，目前成功發表兩篇國際臨床期刊(SCI)論文，首次以客觀實驗驗證「生物光能」的作用如何使不正常的人體皮膚上穴位點產生導電性的正常化作用，亦首次提出經絡具有波動性的實驗觀察結論。另外，針對「生物光能」的診療方式，提出可以利用臨床壓痛點(trigger points)、循經感傳以及利用良導絡儀器(皮膚電阻和電流之左右共二十四穴位點測量儀)，來選擇慢性疾病患者有效生物能治療位置與方式，而目前仍有多篇相關論文投稿中。經過了長達十年和完成超過百種不同的單項種類實驗驗證後，加上二十多篇基礎科學和基礎醫學期刊發表後，我們總結了「生物能陶瓷材料」的特點，包括它具有獨特的物理波傳遞性，可藉由光波、聲波和水波的穿透，把材料可以產生對水、血液、細胞液和組織液的氫鍵弱化，可讓「生物能陶瓷材料」的功能產生後續性的再強化，促進了微血液循環和其他分子醫學能驗證的效應。

「生物光能儀」與「生物能共振儀」針對組織液的水與血液產生作用，具有「生物能量記憶性」、「生物能量人體穿越性」和「生物能量隔空傳遞性」。儀器開發之所以有如此進展，先要追溯三位科學家的貢獻。在 1990 代期間，中國大陸張維波博士提出「經絡是一種存在於組織

間質(interstitial)中、具有低流阻性質的、能夠運行組織液、化學物質和物理量的多孔介質通道」。這假說稱作「經絡的低流阻通道」理論，張維波博士等對這一假說進行了一系列動物實驗驗證。透過放射同位素實驗，通過對小型豬皮膚上，類似人體上的低流阻點下之組織液傳播性的研究，發現循行於經絡的低流阻通道基本位於皮下組織，一般位於脂肪層與肌肉層的結合部位。他們發現，組織液通道除了有連接毛細血管到淋巴管的功能，也有連接組織和組織的功能，許多短小的組織液通道互相溝通形成大通道。這結果啟發了我，就是因為「生物能陶瓷材料」產生對水、血液、細胞液和組織液的氫鍵弱化的功能，所以「生物能陶瓷材料」可以產生對這種低流阻通道之流動促進，鼓勵讓我在二年多前申請與主持台灣科技部研究計劃，來進行傳統醫學實驗，而很快就有了極驚人收穫。

另一方面，以故的英國心血管循環生理學家麥當努醫師(D.A McDonald) 於 1960 年代利用儀器發現了心臟跳動和脈搏在動脈傳導時，是可以利用傅利葉分析(Fourier analysis) ，分解成多個諧波頻率(harmonic wave frequencies)。而根據台灣物理學家王唯工教授的研究，人類心臟平均跳動只需要消耗 1.5 至 1.8 瓦功率，對照於仍在實驗階段的「人功心臟」卻需要消耗數十瓦功率才來維持最基本血液循環；有趣的是，人類心臟能夠成功推動血球經過總長度達十二萬公量長的微血

管來供應細胞氧氣供應，其效率之高是無法想像的，王唯工教授靈活利用血液生理學家麥當努醫生的心臟跳動和脈搏諧波頻率理論，提出動脈與人體器官共振理論，認為各諧波頻率與各個對應器官行成共振，才能推動最有效率的微血液流動。他指出，心臟產生對動脈血管壁上的振波，依不同的振動頻率傳送至全身各部位與器官而產生共振，促進了微血液循環至該區域。他進一步指出中國中醫理論的所謂「十二經絡」，各自對應源自心臟打出來的振動頻率所分解成的諧波頻率。當老化或疾病產生過程時，微血液循環至各器官是不斷下降。如某器官頻率偏移，則局部血流不足，血液就沒有力量進入微血管，所以此器官就因共振不足而缺血、缺氧、缺乏營養及抵抗力，進而代謝之廢物累積，久而久之，百病由此而生。參透了以上理論，「生物光能儀」與「生物能共振儀」的應用，經由選擇不同頻率，促成或加強動脈血管和相對應器官產生共振，透過被傳遞於光波、聲波和水波的生物能量，帶入體內老化和病態器官組織上，創造出一個促進微循環的良好環境，幫忙補救在老化和生病過程中，動脈與人體器官頻率共振不足的問題；同時，可以以科學理論驗證出 2500 年前成書的「黃帝內經」所言：「通則不痛，不通則痛」(可以詮釋為「共振良好會健康，共振不良會生病」)。「生物光能儀」與「生物能共振儀」的應用，針對單一穴位、單一經絡多穴位或多條經絡之照射與頻率共振，能恢

復血液流動暢順，加強微循環，可作為治療慢性疾病之手段，同時成為一個全新的醫療概念。目前「生物光能儀」與「生物能共振儀」已經在衛生福利部台北醫院放射科和台北醫學大學傳統醫學部門診服務病患。

「生物能陶瓷材料」科技的應用成果，包括血糖控制，中風後的康復，失眠和偏頭痛（慢性交感神經系統紊亂）等問題。當結合傳統醫學理論後，其應用更是潛力無窮。另外，經由臨床觀察，我們基本驗證出一半以上傳統中醫所提到的十二經絡，可以與特定諧波頻率產生客觀共振，可在病人身上產生能量傳導現象。

總結以上，我們首次大膽的提出，東西方傳統醫學(包括中國經絡和古代印度人體氣輪學說)，其實是可以用物理學來解釋的。基本上，都是源自於心跳脈搏的物理波動共振現象，

心臟跳動與脈搏週期波動下，在身體固定體積內，形同共振箱內所產生的駐波（Standing wave），而駐波所產生的一系列波腹(Antinodes)就對應其相關的一系列節點(nodes)(請看圖示)；透過節點串連後，各相連節點位置上的組織液(interstitial fluid)，會受到波腹波動之不斷推動，促進了微流道的液態流動，這個微流道很可能是古代中國人發現的經絡通道(Meridian)；而相關的波腹的形成，很可能反映了古代印度所發現的人體氣輪(Chakra)。

生物能陶瓷材料利用光激發（PLB）的效果
運用在中大腦動脈閉塞（MCAO）大鼠的試驗研究

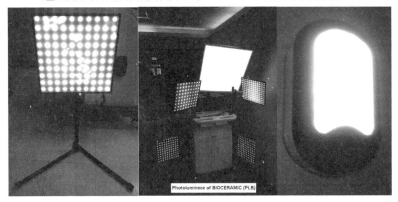

Photoluminece of BIOCERAMIC (PLB)

生物光能儀器

　　這項研究目的是利用生物能陶瓷材料光激發
(PLB:Photoluminence of BIOCERAMIC)的效果運於對
中風的助益，藉由已梗塞性腦中風缺血的動物來做實
驗。記錄缺血性心肌梗塞大鼠在跑步機上的速度和比較
利用生物能陶瓷材料治療後運動能力的改變。實驗統計
結果顯示經由 PLB 照射後能提高運動的速度，且提升
肌肉耐力調控並減少肌肉疲勞，實驗組與對照組 P ＜
0.05。實驗證實生物能陶瓷材料的治療對於改善腦缺血
大鼠的研究很有幫助。

前言：

根據統計國人十大死因中，腦血管疾病歷年來都居高不下。缺血性中風是一種異質性疾病，有各種風險因素。它會導致神經功能的突然喪失，造成腦部有些區域的血液輸送中斷，腦組織得不到足夠的血液供應，而缺乏氧氣及所需的營養素，導致腦組織細胞受損甚至壞死的情形，並且造成身體的殘疾。在我們以前的研究表明了不同的性質和生物效應的生物能陶瓷（高效能陶瓷粉末發射遠紅外線照射），生物能陶瓷材料根據其特點的生物效應，非電離電磁輻射[1]、非線性光子晶體[2]和光激發[3,4]，利用"光激發效應'PLB的概念相結合的生物陶瓷材料（一種發出高性能的紅外線的光子晶體）和可見光光譜的影響。能幫助患者促進微循環[5]和鈣依賴細胞系中的促進一氧化氮增強鈣依賴的一氧化氮合酶[6,7]和鈣調蛋白的上調，也被證明能激活副交感神經系統，這可能會有助於亞極量運動[8]後體能、心臟和呼吸速率恢復的提升。我們希望證實PLB可能有益於中風大鼠的顯著的幫助，利用缺血性梗塞後的動物來做實驗，利用跑步機來鍛鍊大鼠並且記錄，紀載改變速度和比較評估中大腦動脈閉塞(MCAO)大鼠的運動能力。

材料與方法：

生物陶瓷材料的光激發（PLB）利用可見光源的發光二極管（LED），控制照明在 450 ± 50 lux，無需額外的熱效應影響。動物模型實驗：10 隻大鼠（ 200 克; N = 10 ），利用 4-0 手術尼龍縫線置入大鼠內頸動脈(ICA)阻塞中大腦動脈(MCA)，直到管腔內 MCA 供應受阻，取出手術尼龍縫線並且將大鼠縫合，讓血液造成再灌流造成受損。經由 MCAO 手術程序後有 3 隻於 24 小時內死亡，其餘初期出現短暫性神經功能受損，所有腦缺血大鼠幾乎恢復一般的外觀。為了確定腦損傷後大鼠缺血過程，為牠們安排隧道迷宮測試實驗以確定遭受缺血性腦損傷，利用 PLB 加入迷宮實驗，也證實使用 PLB 對於 MCAO 可以縮短迷宮時間。在此次研究中選擇之前參與過迷宮實驗 3 大鼠(N=3)，餵養於籠子裡，溫度 23°C ± 2。MCAO 大鼠於跑步機上做測試，速度分別為 10、20、30、40、50、60、HIGH 和 MAX 速度，從起點到終點每個速度分別跑 3 次，跑完所有速度後整個流程才算結束，若無法達成則算失敗，每實驗一次都必須間隔 24 小時為大鼠休息時間。分別記錄 MCAO 大鼠於跑步機上從原點跑到終點所花費的時間並且計算出每秒所能跑的距離，未照光為對照組，照光後為實驗組。比較對照組與實驗組經由 PLB 照光

後探討速度可否能提升。另外，評估 PLB 照光後是否可以改善肌肉疲勞恢復的實驗，對照組於跑步機跑完整個流程後，休息 30 分鐘合併照光後再跑完整個流程為實驗組，藉此評估肌肉疲勞恢復是否有幫助。

結論：

根據 MCAO 大鼠於跑步機實驗統計結果，針對實行 PLB 照光後速度可否提升，經由平均速率顯示(fig. 1-3)，大鼠 3 號未實行照光發現在跑步機上，跑步速度越來越遲緩到最後到高速時無法往前甚至被拖著走，呈現精疲力盡的狀態；經由 PLB 照光後整個流程皆可以完成，更具意義在高速時可以達成(fig.1)，平均速率 4.07±7.05 cm/s。大鼠 4 號與 8 號、於最高速度時，實驗組與對照組差異雖然不大，但在最大速度時兩者差異性極大，平均速率分別為 27.47±1.03 cm/s、22.54±21.11 cm/s，對照組與實驗組 $p < 0.05$。評估肌肉疲勞度恢復實驗中，原先對照組無法達成甚至失敗，但經由 PLB 照光後先前無法達到的速度都可以完成，甚至超越原先的對照組的平均速率(fig. 4-6)，大鼠 3 號最高速度的平均速率為 6.11±8.04 cm/s、4 號、8 號最大速度的速率各別為 27.47±1.03 cm/s、47±3.04 cm/s，對照組與實驗組 $p < 0.05$，實驗證實生物能陶瓷材料的治療，有助於提升運動速度與肌肉疲勞度恢復，對於改善

腦缺血大鼠的研究很有幫助。

討論：

本次實驗中，額外利用杜普勒超音波血流儀來測量
MCAO 大鼠頸動脈血流，測量動脈平均血流速度
（MN）與最大頻譜峰值（PK），比較運動前後、PLB
照光前後與運動的差異性，預先假設會有顯著差異性；
但結果顯示在實驗中特異性不高並無顯著差異性，p＞
0.05，與先前假設推論不相同，此實驗測量方法仍需要
再加以討論和探討其問題所在。

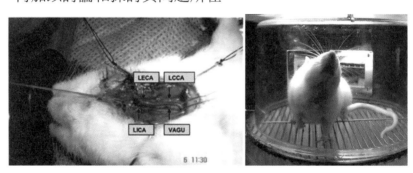

左圖:手術中風老鼠　右圖:生物光能照手術中風老鼠

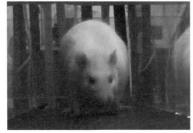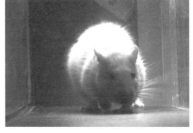

沒有照(左) 與 有照生物光能(右) 的運動中風老鼠

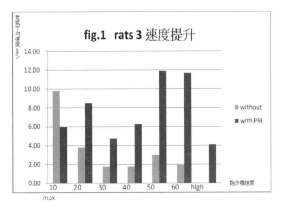

fig.1 rats 3 速度提升

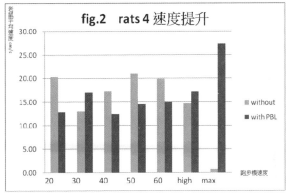

fig.2 rats 4 速度提升

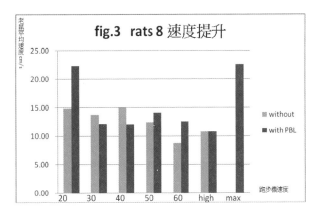

fig.3 rats 8 速度提升

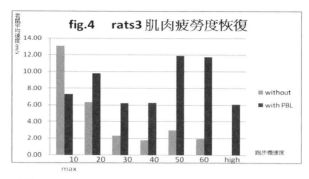

fig.4　rats3 肌肉疲勞度恢復

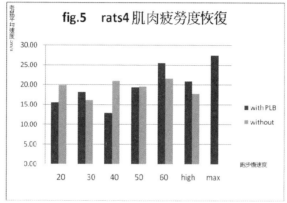

fig.5　rats4 肌肉疲勞度恢復

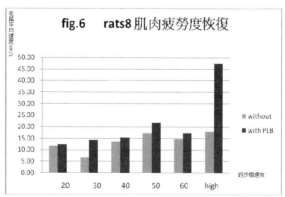

fig.6　rats8 肌肉疲勞度恢復

<Photoluminescence of Bioceramic Materials (PLB) as a Complementary and Alternative Therapy for Diabetes> 已發表在美國醫學期刊 <Diabetes and Metabolism>

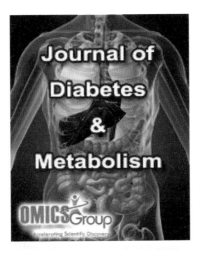

以下為中文內容

生物能陶瓷材料利用光激發（PLB）的效果運用在糖尿病細胞/動物/人體的試驗研究

亞洲和非洲的糖尿病超過西方國際。糖尿病是患者增加和國家經濟的一個重大的財政負擔。此外，終身降糖治療和藥物耐受性，必須尋求非藥物替代療法，以減少抗糖尿病藥物的要求。

生物光能的研究採用了細胞模型，動物模型和臨床試驗，用於作為一個夏目漱石目標，控制在糖尿病患者的高血糖和糖尿。

糖尿病的典型症狀是三多一少，指多飲、多尿、多食、消瘦。患者水分流失過多，發生細胞內脫水，刺激口渴中樞，飲水量和飲水次數都增多以補充水分。糖尿病的症狀還有排尿越多，飲水也越多，形成正比關係；糖尿病人血糖濃度增高，體內不能被充分利用，特別是腎小球濾出而不能完全被腎小管重吸收，以致形成滲透性利尿，出現多尿。血糖越高，排出的尿糖越多，尿量也越多，這也是糖尿病的症狀。消瘦主要是消耗過大所致；由於胰島素不足，機體不能充分利用葡萄糖，使脂肪和蛋白質分解加速來補充能量和熱量。其結果使體內碳水化合物、脂肪及蛋白質被大量消耗，再加上水分的流失，病人體重減輕、形體消瘦，嚴重者體重可下降數十斤，以致疲乏無力，精神不振。

糖尿病是一種慢性、低發炎性疾病。多種因素刺激下，環氧化酶 (COX-2) 在胰島及多種組織中呈現高表現量。它透過與各種發炎因子，如 NF-κB、PGE 等相互作用，對相應組織產生作用，從而促進了糖尿病併發症的發生和發展，包括腎病變、視網膜病變、神經病變、心臟病變等。COX-2 可能為預防和治療糖尿病併發症提供新的思路。此外，研究一致表明患有糖尿病後

體內的一氧化氮活性降低。無論是 I 型還是 II 型糖尿病都有此情形，目前還未完全了解糖尿病患者體內一氧化氮含量降低的機制。一種可能的原因是酸中毒，由於糖尿病主要的機能失常表現是將糖轉化成能量的能力降低；結果造成體內的酸細胞可能抑制一氧化氮的產生，或者耗盡人體內儲存的一氧化氮。另一個可能原因是糖尿病自身導致的破壞性過程，它產生的自由基導致一氧化氮以越來越快的速率被破壞或失去活性。一氧化氮的減少會破壞血管的內皮細胞功能，使血管造成異常收縮，也使血小板容易發生凝集，進而產生血塊阻塞血管，造成更多血管病變；從而引發血液循環不良、心臟病、腎臟病變、眼睛視網膜受損、手指和腳趾的知覺降低（末梢神經病變）以及傷口癒合速度減慢或能力減退等。

此外，在先前的研究亦指出生物光能促進微循環及使血管擴張，並可用於治療血管相關的疾病。本團隊對於生物光能的各研究結果均證明生物陶瓷材料經由弱化水分子氫鍵，影響包括組織液、細胞液與血液並增加擴散，同時增加細胞內外的份子傳遞與內循環。此機制推斷亦有助於帶動葡萄糖傳遞與代謝，同時強化細胞排出毒素和代謝廢物，有利於提高細胞從血液中吸收氧氣的效率。本團隊亦已發表於多篇醫學期刊論文並取得專利，其中證實能促進微循環、促進傷口修復、影響細胞

一氧化氮、攜鈣蛋白與抗氧化能力、降低耗氧量，並能抑制發炎因子如 COX-2、PGE2、緩和疼痛、抒解壓力，調節交感/副交感神經之間交互作用

根據我們在台北醫學大學放射學科的最新研究，經過生物光能治療，可以提升葡萄糖於細胞膜之穿越擴散，帶來糖尿病大鼠糖尿的顯著減少，亦同時降低 95％以上的人類糖尿病患空腹血糖。

通過我們的數據相結合，回顧過去的文章中，我們發現，生物光能治療能促進葡萄糖通過氫鍵減弱和一氧化氮（NO）提升的相關機制，增強的物理擴散力，使血液中過高的葡萄糖穿過細胞膜來成功運輸。在未來，生物光能可能更具有臨床應用的作用，改善高血糖和改善糖尿病相關併發症。

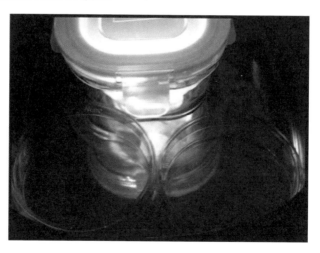

生物光能改善糖尿病相關細胞實驗

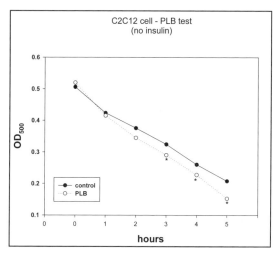

結果顯示細胞外之糖分往細胞內移動

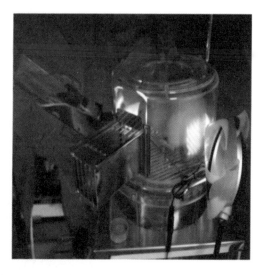

生物光能改善糖尿病相關動物實驗

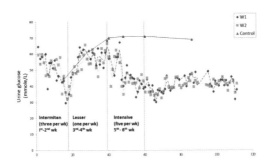

結果顯示動物糖尿改善

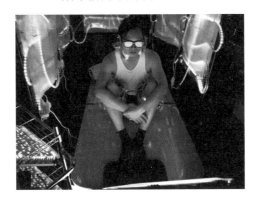

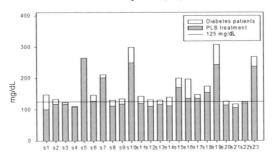

(上)生物光能改善糖尿病相關人體實驗

(下)結果顯示人體血糖照光後下降

無痛針灸，打通經絡

「**生物光能**」具有針對組織液水與血液的「**生物能量記憶性**」、「**生物能量人體穿越性**」和「**生物能量隔空傳遞性**」。「**生物光能**」是「**生物能陶瓷材料**」的延伸，除了具有原來材料的各項特徵外，是「**創新**」、「**超越**」的「**新生命能量**」，更開闢了一些新的應用價值。在經絡穴位的應用上，首先是經絡已被證明是組織液的水性微通道，「生物光能」在「水」的能量轉移上，因為立即產生了氫鍵弱化，以至於瞬間起發「水」的波動性，流動性增加。「生物光能」的應用，有利於解決經絡「水」通道不暢通所產生的生理功能障礙。另外，經絡穴位是光的良導通道，因此，利用「生物光能」配合深層穿越的可見紅光成為新光針療法，不只避免了針灸進針時的疼痛、減少用「針」侵入皮膚時可能感染的疑慮，新光針療法的操作性更是方便，簡單化。以「生物光能」新光針療法的單一穴位、單一經絡多穴位和多條經絡或多穴位照射是一種能量醫學的突破。

「生物能陶瓷材料」和「生物光能」對於「含氯自來水」所產生的除氯效果是檢測生物能量的指標之一：

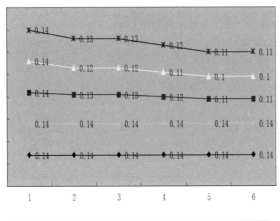

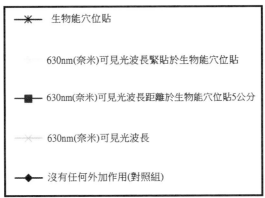

　　「**生物光能**」照射於不含生物光能作用含氯自來
水，結果表明，利用 630nm(奈米)可見光波長緊貼於生
物能穴位貼，使水中餘氯下降量比任一個實驗組和對照
組都低，「**生物光能**」加強了原有「**生物能陶瓷材料**」
的效果。

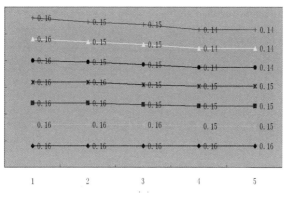

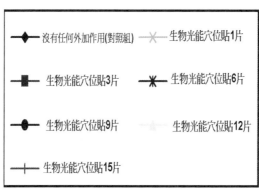

「**生物光能**」穴位貼 *(630nm(奈米) 可見光波長緊貼於生物能穴位貼)* 照射於 含氯自來水，結果表明，增加「生物光能」穴位貼的數量有加強了水中除氯的效果的趨勢。

生物能共振 (BIOCERAMIC Resonance)引發 '身體感覺效應' 和不同心臟跳動諧波頻率所產生駐波有關

介紹

根據我們公佈的數據，生物陶瓷材料已被證明對氫鍵有減弱作用和改變水的液體特性。也證明了它的作用在不同的細胞實驗，動物實驗和人體試驗中，特別是促進微循環。生物能共振是一種新型生物陶瓷的應用技術。根據我們的未公開的數據和觀察，聲頻能夠執行和提高生物陶瓷材料的物理特性，通過很長的距離，並在人體內穿透組織。生物能共振為使用特定的聲波頻率的節拍與生物陶瓷材料一起結合的技術。

我們回顧了頻率的影響，以前的文章和研究，以便為我們自己的研究選擇更好地合適的頻率。我們發現拉斯穆森(G. Rasmussen)的研究已經提到全身振動暴露在一個頻率範圍為 1～20Hz 中得出最顯著的影響。我們採用了其中間值---10Hz 的聲波頻率節拍作為第一個研究對象。

在 1960 年代，D.A.博士 McDonald 和他的同事們發現，每個心臟搏動傳播出的動脈搏的頻率可以透過傅里葉分析被分解為多個諧波頻率。在連接到這一點，台

灣物理學家王唯工教授建議，每個人不同的原始心跳諧波頻率，產生與不同的內部器官之共振，進而與體內特定器官和血管床之間發生的共振模式。王教授還提出，共振頻率的最重要功能是幫助微血流中的血液進入特定器官。根據他的發表，如果心臟跳動保持固定在每分鐘72 次，王教授仍為這些諧波頻率被發現在 1.2Hz 至 13.2 赫茲（表1）的範圍內。

我們研究的目的是觀察 "生物能共振'產生與心臟跳動特定諧波頻率共振的聲波節拍,是否產生人體的某種效應。

諧波數 （HW）	1st HW	2nd HW	3rd HW	4th HW	5th HW	6th HW	7th HW	8th HW	9th HW	10th HW	11th HW (假設)	12th HW (假設)
赫茲估計 (以心臟跳 動率在 72/分鐘)	1.2	2.4	3.6	4.8	6.0	7.2	8.4	9.6	10.8	12	13.2	能量總合

表1：根據固定在每分鐘72次標準心跳基線相關的各諧波頻率

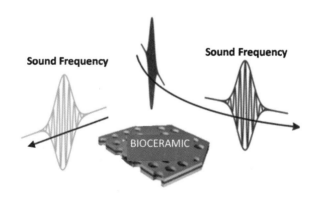

圖 1 生物能(BIOCERAMIC)共振概念

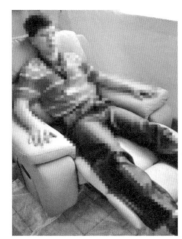

生物能復康使
用生物能共振

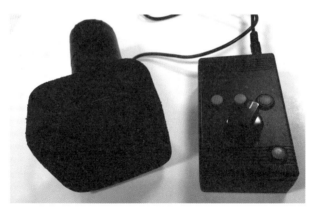

圖 2a＆B：醫療用生物能大共振設備和小生物能共振

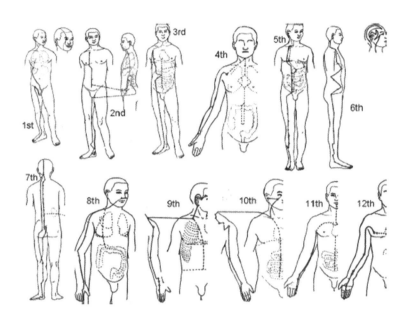

圖 3：不同的諧波頻率(1st 到 12th)與身體相對應的路線圖

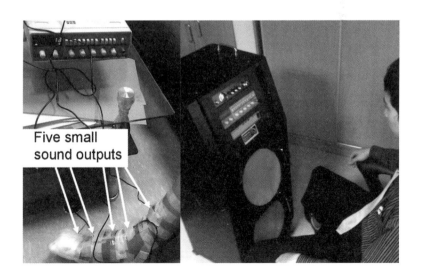

Five small
sound outputs

圖 4：採用小生物能共振輸出（左，4A）；使用大生物能共
　　　振輸出（右，圖 4b）

結果

生物能共振作用在 10Hz 的人體實驗結果

在實驗過程中，二十位實驗參考者，身體有主觀感
覺效應達十六位，他們分別記錄有皮膚上，皮下組織或
及肌肉群不同程度的感受，其描述和數據現示於表 2。

性別	記錄區域	根據心臟跳動，相對應的諧波頻率數（HF）	備註
女性	雙邊前臂腹面	12th	
女性	雙邊小腿和大腿內側	1st	
男性	背部中線	未能分類	
男性	雙邊小腿和大腿之外側	6th	
女性	右邊小腿和大腿外側	6th	
男性	後邊頭皮上依靠右	6th	之前出血性中風右上肢和下肢無力
女性	左邊大腳趾背面	3rd	

男性	右上肢背側	8th	之前因結腸癌接受外科治療
女性	右上肢背側	8th	右側急性肩痛
女性	右小腿和大腿的外側面	6th	
女性	雙邊前臂腹面內側	11th	
女性	右小腿和大腿外側面	6th	
女性	雙邊前臂腹面內側	11th	
女性	右上肢背面	8th	右側急性肩痛
男性	雙邊小腿和大腿內側面	1st	
男性	右小腿和大腿外側	6th	右側頸部疼痛

表 2: 生物能共振輸入之聲音節拍頻率：約 10Hz

生物能共振在不同的聲音輸出頻率的結果

生物能共振通過使用不同特定頻率，記錄了 17 位測試者不同身體感覺效應。按照圖 3 所顯示心跳數的特定諧波頻率，透過感覺效應找出共振區路線(road map)，它表示特定諧波頻率的特定位置點。數據和說明列於表 3。

性別	生物能共振來源	每分鐘的心率	建議共振頻率	最有效的諧波頻率（HF）數	匹配或不匹配	備註
男性	小共振	70	7-8	6th	匹配	
女性	小共振	89	3.4	3rd	匹配	
男性	小共振	72	3.6	6th	不匹	

性別	生物能共振來源	每分鐘的心率	建議共振頻率	最有效的諧波頻率（HF）數	匹配或不匹配	備註
					配	
女性	小共振	70	3.6	6th	不匹配	小腿疼痛
女性	小共振	85	1.4	1st	匹配	虛弱
女性	小共振	80	6	5th	匹配	
女性	小共振	72	12	10th	匹配	
男性	小共振	65	3	3rd,	匹配	已接受脾切除術
男性	小共振	72	6	5th	匹配	
男性	小共振	80	5	6th	不匹配	
女性	大共振	73	7	6th	匹配	
女性	大共振	72	7	6th	匹配	
M 男性	大共振	71	7	6th	匹配	
男性	大共振	73	7	6th	匹配	

性別	生物能共振來源	每分鐘的心率	建議共振頻率	最有效的諧波頻率（HF）數	匹配或不匹配	備註
女性	大共振	74	6	5th	匹配	面部不自主運動
男性	大共振	72	1.2	1st	匹配	
男性	大共振	73	6	5th	匹配	

表 3：實驗 2 的結果

　　根據第一個實驗中，我們注意到，女性受試者比男性多出四成，更能明白生物能共振產生對身體感覺效應。最常見的身體感覺效應的位置被發現是在第 6 諧波頻率上（約 37.5％），這比第二和第三等位，分別是第 8 諧波頻率（13.75％）和 11 諧波頻率（12.5％）的總和更為頻繁。

　　在第二個實驗中，所需生物能大共振來代替生物能小共振才產生身體感覺效應的百分比為 41％。結果表明以心臟跳動諧波頻率來預期感覺效應在身體上特定位置超過 82.3％是匹配的。而不匹配的身體感覺效應之心臟跳動諧波頻率都是第 6 次諧波頻率。此外，我們還觀察到參與第二個實驗中的幾個受試者顯示身體感覺有

"跳躍效應"，意思是感覺出現在不是預期的中醫經絡路線上，就是其它經絡路線位置上。

討論

如所提到的，生物陶瓷材料和"生物能共振"儀器對組織中之流動體液、水和血液的氫鍵，觀察到有顯著影響的現象。為了討論本研究的成果，應該提及三名科學家的貢獻。在 1990 年代，張維波博士團隊進行了一系列針對穴位和經絡的探索性研究，利用放射同位素測量動物體內組織間液壓力，其結果是，一個連接定點的分形通道的存在得到確認，是一種低水壓阻力通道，同時認為宅是中國傳統醫學中描述的 "經絡'。經絡是組織間質流體動液體是，為連接血管，淋巴管和細胞間的空間;然而，現代生理學沒有太重視組織間質液，一些臨床醫生更辯論組織液是否能實際自由地流動。張維波博士團隊的實驗結果表明，較低的水阻力通道（LHRC）的實際存，是沿中國傳統醫藥中描述的經絡位置。較低的水阻力通道（LHRC）的發現提供生理醫學較完整來解釋經絡，和流動通道可以通過放射同位素軌跡的移動來進行定位。另一方面，由於生物陶瓷材料(BICOERAMIC)的主要作用是產生的液體氫鍵減弱，因此它可能產生於由張維波博士所提到的低阻力流體通道的實際影響。

在 20 世紀 60 年代期間，D.A. McDonald 麥當勞醫生和他的團隊發現，利用傅立葉分析傳播動脈脈搏的每個心跳頻率可以分解成多個諧波頻率。王唯工教授提出，心血管生理學的問題，並聲稱，心臟跳動的平均功耗只有 1.5～1.8 瓦，功率太小，無法解釋其實現的對紅血球細胞的有效運輸能力。相反，人造心臟使用超過 50 瓦的功率消耗才能保持基本的血液循環，但仍然不適合於一般的心臟移植，無法使人長期存活。其實，人的心臟每天成功完成，通過毛細血管網絡，達到十二公里長，所推動血液流動和輸送氧氣供給細胞。根據王唯工教授等人先前建立和完成之一系列體外和體內動物實驗，是使用由麥當勞醫生提到心臟跳動脈搏的諧波頻率理論。王認為動脈和器官之間有具體的頻率，人體內有如存在對應於螺旋彈簧結構，形成鏈接在一起各器官共振模式，按各次諧波的頻率形成共鳴，共振的原因是幫助促進和保持微血液循環流動的有效性。要注意的是，心跳產生振動傳播沿動脈壁和血液流動，這在某種程度上取決於，不同傳輸頻率於不同特定血管床和器官產生特定頻率共振。他進一步指出，所謂的中國傳統醫學"十二經脈"理論，就是從心臟跳動脈搏波分解出一系列諧波頻率。在老化過程和病理過程中，會使微血液循環下降，在缺乏局部血流量是無法有效推動含氧血液到各種血管床的組織和器官。換句話說，由特定動脈脈搏

波之間的諧波共振變差開始，對應於特定的血管床和器官之組織開始缺氧，營養缺乏，免疫削弱，積累毒素等所述結果，隨著時間的惡化狀況下，帶來的不同的疾病。生物能共振基於上述理論，選擇特定的頻率的應用，可以創建輸入頻率和血管床和器官對應的特定的心臟脈搏諧波頻率之間的共振，與生物陶瓷材料原本的液體氫鍵弱化和促進微血液循環在人體的影響結合。根據這個概念，生物能共振與特定的輸入頻率共振，有助於加強動脈和器官之微血液循環，從而創造了有利的環境，以幫助減緩衰老過程和疾病的功能障礙。此外，通過臨床觀察，使用生物能共振裝置，超過一半的參與者驗證出身體的特定共振通道路線感覺，這種現象也被稱為沿經絡感傳現象（Propagating sensation along meridian），並已報導在我們之前發表的醫學期刊上。

我們進一步發現，上述觀察到的中醫經絡現象，本身可以通過 "駐波" (Standing wave)的物理概念來解釋。正如我們所知，駐波是保持在一個恆定位置的波形運動。這種現象的原因，是兩個以相反方向運動的波形重疊所產生。 "駐波" 在介質中以特定頻率共振之後，建立出節點（靜止的點）和波腹（脈動波）持續位於相同的介質位置上。不同次諧波的頻率從心臟跳動脈波開始，來發動和振動，通過動脈血管進行傳播（圖5）。當脈搏波到達在主動脈及髂總動脈分岔，部分脈

搏波向後行進回到主動脈。最後，產生相同的諧波頻率波形重疊，互相干擾共振產生"駐波"，而這情況也發生在較小的動脈（圖5）。

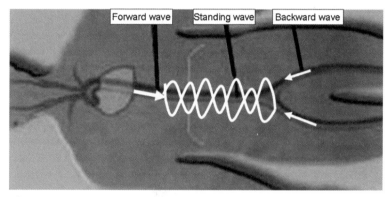

圖5：正向和反向傳輸波，碰撞在一起，干擾後形成駐波

　　以立體思維，波腹的恆定的振動，產生在結點上的推力，形成組織液通道的流動作用，持續的心跳產生一系諧波與所屬"駐波"，保持流體運動順暢，形成了中醫所謂的經絡（圖6）。

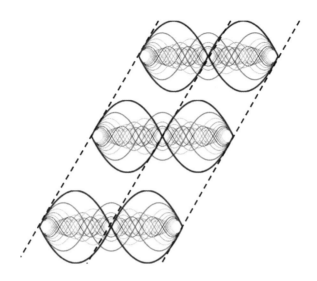

圖 6：我們推論，在駐波上各節點連接成虛線，通過波腹推
　　　力，產生對位於節點上組織液，形成組織液通道的流
　　　動作用，代表中醫經絡

　　要解釋為什麼實驗中最多身體感覺效應，是在第 6
次諧波的頻率，我們認為這個頻率（約 7.0-8.0Hz），
與舒曼共振(Schumann resonance)的頻率範圍相似。
舒曼諧振被定義為地表和電離層邊界之間的頻率共振模
式。舒曼共振在不同地理位位置上有一些變化，基本是
大氣層上形成的駐波。這不是一個巧合，舒曼共振的頻
率範圍與靜息狀態下的所有哺乳動物中發現的主要 α 腦
電波節律重疊。在一定條件下，舒曼共振的頻率範圍，
與除特定腦電波產生共鳴。實際上，很多以前觀察到卻

不能解釋的某些心理協調功能，與心理能量信息之傳播都與之有關。因此，我們可以假設，在生物能共振的效應下，心臟跳動之脈搏波的第 6 次諧波的頻率，可能會產生與舒曼共振和 α 腦電波頻率兩者額外的共振，所以可以解釋為什麼第 6 次諧波頻率在身體感覺效應出現更頻繁。在身體感覺效應數的性別差異，可能是男性和女性之間的基本心理活動，各種刺激反應有差異所反映的。我們觀察身體感覺效應的跳躍效果，在我們之前凹發表的數據也同樣顯示經絡之間是有波形流動。總之，我們的研究結果提供行之有效的中醫模式的經絡通道提供科學上驗證。此外，我們認為，這樣的經絡通道可以和從心臟的跳動起源不同的諧波頻率的傳播以及主動脈脈搏形成的 "駐波" 來解釋。這項研究還提供研究人員在科學領域中，有助於解釋一些傳統中國醫學 理論的奧秘。在以下的文章中，我們將介紹生物陶瓷這一新的醫療技術的臨床益處。

2013 年 10 月我們在台北的研究，以主題為<生物光能進行穴道照射，發現循經絡波動現象><Wave-Induced Flow in Meridians Demonstrated Using Photoluminescent Bioceramic Material on Acupuncture Points>，獲得發表在美國「實證替代醫學雜誌」(Evidence-Based Complementary and Alternative Medicine; Volume 2013, Article ID 739293, 11 pages)(梁

庭繼等/Ting Kai Leung el al)

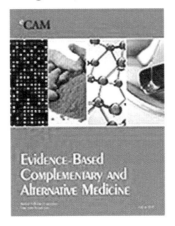

以下為論文摘要:

<前言>

　　經絡穴位針灸的機制仍然知之甚少，但一般認為，經絡導電率(良導絡儀)的測量提供之客觀數據，代表不同的經絡能量。在過去，非侵入性的刺激經絡穴位方法，如熱，電，磁鐵，和雷射等，但都沒有很成功取代侵入性的傳統針灸。生物陶瓷材料--光致發光光能量（PLB）已被證明可以削弱體液氫鍵，並改變水/液體的特性。在這項研究中，我們採用非侵入性的（PLB）技術對經絡穴位照射，試圖檢測其效果，通過使用經絡導電率(良導絡儀)的測量，尋找經絡上的信息，包括經絡穴位的流動特性。

<材料和方法>

我們測量經絡穴位導電率，在 76 例患者中，檢測各種經絡穴位具有極高或極低的電流導電水平，選擇最異常的經絡穴位點。我們應用（PLB）對其經絡穴位點照射 15 分鐘。

<結果>

經絡穴位點經由（PLB）照射 15 分鐘表現出了可靠的互補效應，最低與最高的經絡穴位導電率，返回到或接近正常水平。而特定經絡穴位之間有連動關係存在。

<討論>

基於實驗結果和文獻回顧，我們發現經絡穴位具有流動特質。

我們推論經絡穴位具有流體力學波形，能解釋過去文獻報告的經絡電流傳導性，聲學傳導性、熱傳導性、光傳導性、同位素傳導性和流體傳導性等等。

我們進一步推斷，經絡通道是相互關聯的，經由穴位刺激誘導的經絡通道系統，致使波浪型流動增加，符合過去文獻提出經絡和穴位是人體組織間微液通道的概念。

<結論>

　　我們的數據顯示，經絡穴位點經由（PLB）照射後，異常的經絡穴位點都有電流流動的互補效應，返回到其正常的電流水平，特定經絡之間有相互影響性。在未來，非侵入性的(PLB) 可應用於刺激經絡，可用於調節經絡穴位，達到類似傳統針灸的治療效果。

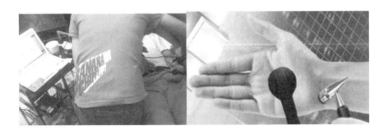

圖　實驗人員正進行良導絡儀測試中

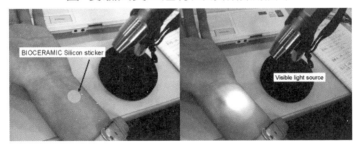

上圖　生物能量矽膠貼於心包經內關穴(左)，即進行生物光能照射(右)

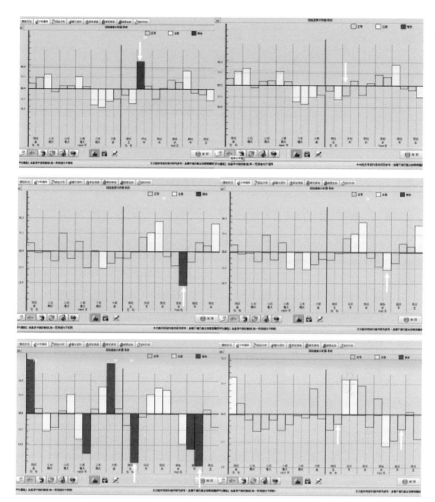

生物光能在特定穴位照射前(左上.左下圖)，照射後(右左上.
右下圖)，實驗人員再進行良導絡儀測試，會發現特定穴位
電流流動的互補效應，返回到其正常的電流水平

134

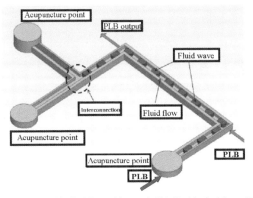

上圖 我們推論: 經絡像捷運線，穴道像其車站，經絡與經
絡之暑可以互通，或不互通

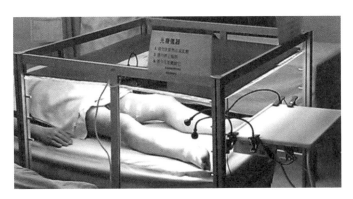

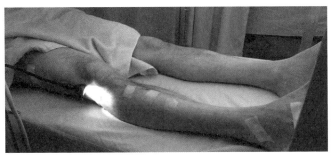

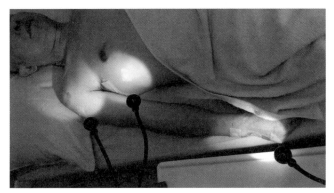

上圖 生物光能循經絡照射

Application of Photoluminescent Bioceramic Material(PLB) for different chronic illnesses by selecting 'Trigger Points' and 'Propagated Sensation along Meridians' (PSM) phenomenon 發表在國際級醫學期刊 Chinese Journal of Integrative Medicine(SCI)

生物光能 Photoluminescent Bioceramic Material （PLB）通過選擇 "壓痛點" 和 "感傳沿經絡' （PSM）現象的應用於不同慢性疾病

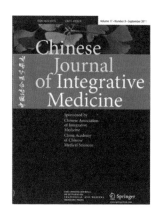

以下為論文摘要：

前言

　　中國傳統醫學中最重要的經典之作 "黃帝內經" 提到："通則不痛，痛則不通"，意思是: 那裡沒有障礙(生病)，就沒有疼痛；那裡有障礙(生病)會有疼痛。中國古代醫生認為存在於人體內的微小通道停滯，是個人疾病產生的原因。健康是需要適當的體內水分流量和生命能量平衡的結果。中國醫學認為通過遍布全身之經絡和氣順利運行才能健康。在中國，針灸已經應用了數千年。亦傳到中國周邊地區，目的為平衡經絡通道，來治療各種急性或慢性疾病。然而今天，由於其侵入性的本質，和難以科學解釋，不為西醫界所普遍接受。氣功，是一種非侵入性治療，廣泛性平衡身心健康，但由於太

費時間才能看到臨床益處。

生物光能（PLB）對經絡通道的作用，通過特定穴位照射，是一項新開發的技術。近年來，生物能陶瓷材料的一系列科研成果，包括物理-化學、物理-生物科學、基礎醫學和臨床科學領域。生物光能具有非侵入性與具有快速作用性的優點。我們利用良導絡儀器之數據分析，我們已經發現生物光能照射前後，PLB 具有能量在經絡使阻塞再次返回正常 流動水平的互補作用。

在這項研究中，我們收集了不同類型的慢性和急性疾病患者，並給予生物光能治療，進行臨床觀察。通過應用"通則不痛，痛則不通"傳統的中國醫學概念，來改善微小的流體通道停滯(經絡不通)，這項研究證明異常阻塞微小的流體通道，可透過良導絡儀器之皮膚電位差異來反映，生物光能照射產生改善。這項研究還有助於我們證明如何選擇 "局部壓痛點'(Trigger points)和 "循經感傳" (Propagated Sensation along Meridians, PSM)現象中的顯示出來，同時幫助找出不同的疾病所對應的異常經絡通道。

結果

我們的實驗結果發現，有 10 名患者接收標準的西方醫學治療但沒有任何顯著改善的病患。他們的病名、相關主訴，和如何選擇生物光能照射穴位以及臨床觀察

（客觀的和主觀的改善），之記錄被列於表 1

有關如何選擇 "觸痛點" 或 "循經感傳" 觀察仔找出相應的異常經絡選擇，列在表 2 中。

有 30%的受試者開始覺得沿著經絡通道傳播的的感覺。儘管是主觀，不能被解釋或歸因於外部熱或疼痛刺激的影響。當中，有兩位受試者明顯在其病情得到改善，包括 "良性面部震顫" 和 "第五腰椎壓迫骨折創傷破壞後截癱" 的案件。他們的疾病持續時間分別為 5 個月和 3 個月。其他病患有不同情況下的主觀和客觀的改善。有 43.8％在臨床改善是客觀的看法。這些當中，下腿或腳水腫是最顯著的客觀改善（100％）。

討論

在這項研究中，我們發現，特定經絡通道透過生物光能照射，具有不同慢性和急性病症有益的結果。但是到現在為止，在醫院和實驗室，利用現代影像和診斷設備仍無法觀察穴位或經絡通道。雖然有 20％的病人由於外傷或手術後截癱，失去皮膚感覺，最終透過其他方法找出相對應穴道/經絡。但在其他 80％的病人中，我們成功地完成了如何選擇 "局部壓痛點'(Trigger points) 和 "循經感傳"（ PSM）現象，來連接出針對病人路線圖(Road map)，反映出經絡通道。生物光能照射因為被證明是一個合理的實證醫學技能。關於臨床觀察，我們

發現的最顯著的改進，主要出現在病程介於亞急性期，就是病發為 3～5 個月後。有關疼痛點，大多數人被發現位於肌肉或組織中，是疼痛的結節。當這種結節被按下（觸診）產生急性疼痛的感覺，被定義為 "壓痛點"。

有趣的是，確定壓痛點的位置，與相傳統的中國醫學穴位的位置之重疊性超過 70％。另一方面，"循經感傳"（PSM）的感覺是一種現象，即沿經絡穴位的刺激，會產生在皮膚相關路徑的感觸，例如移動感覺。"循經感傳"（PSM）的感覺在之前的研究推斷，是神經傳輸與空間的機制或錯覺(volume transmission)與同時亦與組織液中的低阻抗通道旁組織胺之分泌有關，它可以擴張微血管和增加血液灌注和間質流體，同時發送一個連續的可感覺信號，刺激神經系統，該系統可以是覺得身上有"循經感傳"（ PSM）現象。

生物光能之效果是純物理性質為基礎，沒有如進行針灸過程中的組織損傷風險，同時卻產生如同針灸過程中可以感受的 "循經感傳"（ PSM）現象。

根據我們之前的論文發表，要解釋生物光能的有益處和臨床效果，是由於生物光能的照射對經絡通道的基本概念：生物光能治療直接削弱氫鍵和改變組織水的液體特點，誘導或促進沿著經絡通道之流體/水擴散，並因老化或生病致使組織液逐漸停滯。雖然目前的影像科

技仍無法針對經絡的微觀流體通道，作出直接觀察，我們認為這種障礙會被克服，最終隨著技術的進步，生物光能照射的直接效益，以及經絡通道的奧秘將被揭示。我們希望這項工作的公佈後，吸引更多對生物光能科技的支持，並帶來更多有關生物能陶瓷開創性的研究與興趣。

　　總之，我們通過通過選擇"壓痛點"和"感傳沿經絡'（PSM）現象，來選擇合適於病患本身需要的經絡通道，而且在臨床上已被證明是既實用又成功的。這同時驗證了傳統中國醫學理論"通則不痛，痛則不通"之真實性。

表1

疾病	主訴	生病時間	經絡選擇方式	經絡	生物光能照射次數（一個療程為一小時）	客觀或主觀臨床的改善
由於頸脊髓損傷截癱是	嚴重癱瘓夜間背部和下肢疼痛	5年	利用良導絡	膀胱經絡	3週內3個療程	夜間疼痛解除（主觀）
良性的面部震顫	雙側面部不受控制之靜止性震顫	5個月	壓痛點	肝經絡	4週內4個療程	面部震顫完全緩解（客觀）
第五腰椎椎體	(1)截癱和夜間右下肢	3個	壓痛點	膀胱經絡	8週內8個療程	(1)雙邊小腿和腳浮腫

疾病	主訴	生病時間	經絡選擇方式	經絡	生物光能照射次數（一個療程為一小時）	客觀或主觀臨床的改善
壓縮骨折後再創傷引發截癱	疼痛 (2) 雙側小腿和腳浮腫	月		和膽經絡		緩解（客觀） (2) 截癱恢復（客觀）
雙側下肢神經肌肉病	(1) 雙側下肢的大腿感覺與運動力下降 (2) 小腿和腳寒冷感 (3) 夜間抽筋 (4) 左上臂和下臂的疼痛	12年	壓痛點和"循經感傳"（PSM）現象	肝經絡和大腸經絡	6個星期內8個療程	(1) 顯著增加表面溫暖 (2) 雙側下肢的大腿感覺與運動力回增加小腿和腳（客觀） (3) 夜間抽筋痊癒 (4) 左上臂和下臂的疼痛改善（主觀）
腦出血性中風	(1) 右上肢和下肢的半身不遂 (2) 雙側下肢感覺與運動力下降	6年	壓痛點和"循經感傳"（PSM）現象	膽經絡和三焦經絡	7週之內9個療程	雙側下肢感覺與運動力提升（主觀）
後右髖關節和	臀部和下肢疼痛	3年	壓痛點和"循	肝經絡	2週內3個療程	增加右下肢運動力和感

疾病	主訴	生病時間	經絡選擇方式	經絡	生物光能照射次數(一個療程為一小時)	客觀或主觀臨床的改善
股骨創傷性骨折導致運動無力			經感傳"(PSM)現象			覺(主觀)
(1)大腦缺血性中風,導致雙側半身不遂 (2)胸痛,上腹疼痛,大便出血	(1)雙側下肢癱瘓 (2)雙邊小腿和腳浮腫 (3)嗜睡	3年	利用良導絡	膀胱經絡	2週內3個療程	(1)減少水腫(客觀) (2)胸痛,上腹疼痛,大便出血顯著的改善(主觀)
由於鼻部手術的並發症面部震顫	雙側面部肌肉,下頜關節的不隨意運動	6年	壓痛點	膽經絡和肝經絡	5週內10個療程	雙側面部肌肉,下頜關節的不隨意運動略有改善(主觀)
雙側腿和腳的慢性和亞急性	(1)發紅,水腫,雙側小腿和腳的疼痛	1年	壓痛點	肝經絡和膽經	3週內6個療程	雙側下腿和腳水腫消退和發紅改善（客

143

疾病	主訴	生病時間	經絡選擇方式	經絡	生物光能照射次數(一個療程為一小時)	客觀或主觀臨床的改善
炎症	(2) 鎮痛步態			絡		觀)
後顱腦損傷後遺：症面部麻木（右側）	(1) 頭部右頂枕陣發性麻木 (2) 臉麻木	2年來	壓痛點	膽經絡	3週內6個療程	改進右臉麻木（主觀）

表 2

透過壓痛點與 "循經感傳"（PSM）現象來找出不正常之經絡方法	百分比(%)
壓痛點之百分比	80%
"循經感傳"（PSM）現象之百分比	30%
壓痛點與 "循經感傳"（PSM）現象之百分比	30%
壓痛點與 "循經感傳"（PSM）現象都沒有之百分比	20%

攜帶式生物光能共振儀(BIOCERAMIC RESONACE)是由台灣生物能實驗室團隊所研發，生物陶瓷能量至今已經獲得 20 項世界專利與發表 25 篇國際性醫學期刊論文。生物能實驗室的多篇研究論文更被美國哈佛大學、麻省理工大學和麻省總醫院所引用至他們的研究論文中。另一方面，生物能相關產品更獲得日內瓦發明展特別獎與金獎雙料殊榮。

2012年日內瓦國際發明展
特別獎獎盃

2012年日內瓦國際發明展
金牌獎獎牌

2012年科威特中東國際發明展
金牌獎獎牌

2012年科威特中東國際發明展
銅牌獎獎牌

有關生物能陶瓷，生物能陶瓷是一種非游離輻射光譜發射材料，它具有明顯的光致發光特性。先前的研究中我們使用傅立葉變換紅外光譜（FT-IR），對生物能陶瓷照射水發現氫鍵減弱變化。此外，過去發表的研究報告記載了例如被生物陶瓷能處理水之粘度、揮發性、水結晶溫度、表面張力、擴散性、固體顆粒的溶解度，以及乙酸 pH 的變化；結果顯示其粘度和表面張力降低（接觸角實驗），但是在固體顆粒溶解度、結晶水溫度和乙酸的 pH 都增加。結論是由於生陶瓷物能照射水產生氫鍵減弱現象。這一發現驗證過去一系列有關生物陶瓷能的基礎醫學生物學研究，包括對微循環的增強作

用，是因為物理效應所引導。由於水被賦予生命過程中的最重要的部分，在水的氫鍵弱化下，改變水的性質和水團縮小，可以讓生命大環境中的水在不同條件下，以不同的方式表現其特徵。已經証明它能削弱水的氫鍵從而增強微循環。另一方面，體內實驗(in vivo)下，我們發現生物陶瓷能作用有助於正常化不正常之心臟速率和血壓，以及強化心肌收縮。它還顯著減少肌肉僵硬和疼痛的肩頸筋膜炎。生物陶瓷能是通過調節自主神經系統（ANS），經由心臟心率變異性（HRV）測試，證明生物陶瓷能有助於緩解經痛。另一項研究利用心率變異性分析，通過執行連續運動顯示了生物陶瓷能顯著增加了高頻（HF）功率譜，反映生物陶瓷能加強副交感神經。生物光能是建基於生物陶瓷能的特性，加上使用可見光光譜的波長(390 至 750nm)，行成紅外光光譜內的'光激發光'效應，強化前面提到生物陶瓷能所原本產生之物理，生物和物理化學作用，然後傳遞到遠距離或滲透組織的深層。另一方面，生物能共振儀的功能也建基於生物陶瓷能的特徵，經由低頻音波帶動，然後以一定距離傳播或滲透活組織深層產生共振，其擴散力更超越生物光能。通過選擇低頻音波的特殊聲頻率，生物能共振產生的振動與人體不同的組織或器官產生共振。根據我們的研究，生物光能與生物能共振可以應用於中國傳統醫學中，帶來臨床效果。要瞭解生物光能治療儀為何

能

可以應用於中國傳統醫學中，要先知道：“氣為血之帥，血為氣之母”：氣血的運行，保持著相互對立相互依存的關係，氣為陽，是動力；血為陰，是物質基礎。營血在經脈中之所以能不停地運行周流全身，有賴于“氣”作為它的動力。氣行血亦行，氣滯血亦滯，所以說“氣為血帥”。但“氣”必須依賴營血才能發揮作用，所以又有“血為氣母”的說法。它們的關係是，血液營養組織器官而產生機能活動，而機能的正常活動又推動了血液的運行。氣血的運行，也體現了“陰陽互根”的道理。根據台北梁庭繼主任醫師指出，中國傳統醫學所提到的“氣”，就是心跳的各種共振波，能驅使血液循經，血液營養組織器官而產生機能活動，又維持心跳與脈搏位能與動能來運轉循環系統，與推動微血管中帶氧紅血球穿梭細胞周圍，而“氣”的運行，是各組織之共振或是共振效應中的生物能量，此能量尚未普遍被生理科學所定義，但是，參與我們生物能研究的專家都清楚知道，生物能實驗室領先全球，我們不只掌握“氣”---生物能量，而且應用了它。

在台北生物能實驗室，已經完成一系列有關生物光能共振科技在動物和人體試驗(核准編號：IACVCApproval LAC-101-0093、TH-IR0014-0001、TMU-

JIRB201207024 、 TMU-JIRB201210029 、 TMU-IRB-
CRC-02 -08-08 、 TMU-JIRB201007004 和 TMU-
JIRB201105006)。

　　在台北，已在各大醫學大學/醫學中心開辦生物能
醫學門診，包括台北醫學大學附設醫院、輔仁大學醫學
院、衛生福利部台北醫院等。生物光能共振產品與生物
能量產品已經與多家票選為台灣百大品牌合作，例如和

成衛浴 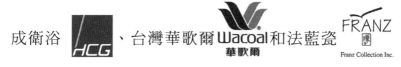 、台灣華歌爾和法藍瓷

等。生物能更席捲全台灣，反應熱烈，廣受好評

　　回顧生物光能共振技巧在治療效果的醫學研究，發
現它能明顯改善失眠、偏頭痛、顏面神經顫抖症等自律
神經系統紊亂所引發的病症；明顯改善失眠；糖尿病的
血糖控制；改進中風後的運動能力； 下肢腫痛(包括血
管發炎)。利用中國傳統經絡醫學的概念，透過作用中
國傳統十二經絡的共振，進而能預防與治療百病，更進
一步証明經絡共振理論的真實性。我們認為，生物陶瓷
能的新技術在替代性治療和中國傳統醫學應用上，具有
廣闊的前景和價值。

三·儀器功能

生物光能輸出：主要針對全身微血液循環，有效改善失眠、偏頭痛、顏面神經顫抖症等自律神經系統紊亂所引發的病症；改善糖尿病的血糖控制；改進中風後的運動能力； 下肢腫痛(包括血管發炎)，另有淡化皮膚黑色素等效果。請直接靠近患處使用照光，一次使用時間十五分鐘以上，不限次數。

生物能共振輸出：輸出脈衝頻率之生物能波形，透過可調控之生物能共振頻率來作用身體十二經絡，使生物能量補充至共振不良的某特定十二經絡上。使用時身體儘量靠近儀器，請先調至最高之生物能共振頻率，從高頻開始感受，如果身體某處慢慢有特別的痛或麻感(循經感傳現象)，代表這個生物能共振頻率已有效產生該處所屬經絡之共振，同時代表該處所屬經絡共振不良，需要補充生物能量。但如果沒感覺，嘗試往下調動，有點像在使用傳統調頻收音機來找電台播放一樣。一般而言，有百分之 70 的人會感覺到身體某處慢慢有特別的痛或麻感(循經感傳現象)，但仍然有百分之 30 天生就不會感覺到，如果沒有找到，就調到最高頻率，繼續使用生物能共振。另外，

如能配合使用生物能穴位貼，貼合在穴位和經絡線上(包括壓痛點和阿是穴)，會達到最好之效果。

針對以中國傳統醫學為概念的使用方式如下：

四‧儀器使用方式與學理

先尋找疾病相對應經絡之方式

利用「通則不痛，不通則痛」原理尋找疾病相對應經絡

(1)壓痛點(trigger point)

中醫認為，「通則不痛，不通則痛」。捏著肉痛，那就說明經絡不通，道理就這麼簡單。經絡不通，人體會發出某些信號，人體是非常敏感的，如果經絡不通，就會發出很多不舒服的信號來求救。現代醫學認為壓痛點是位於肌肉纖維結節，可能是骨骼肌過度激活的斑點，與肌肉纖維過度繃緊有關。在皮膚肌肉或組織中找到急性疼痛的感覺，當這些結節在觸診壓下觸發疼點。而且引起疼痛症狀輻射。

皮膚觸痛點過去是一種不明原因的疼痛，從這些點局部壓痛的輻射到更廣泛的領域。當可靠地識別牽涉痛的哪一個位置與別處皮膚觸痛點聯動疼痛線。目前在相同病變的不同個體患者，發現是類似的位置。有趣的是，相比中國傳統醫學穴位的位置，已被確定觸發點分佈相同度超過 70 ％。根據我們在台北的經驗，當病情

已經達到某種嚴重度，病人的某些地方，會產生皮膚觸痛點的選擇來連接對應於經絡的路線圖，如果能夠一邊找出皮膚觸痛點，同時對照經絡路線圖來找出可能的經絡(例如:心包經)，之後就可以把能量片貼合在經絡路線上，進行光照。

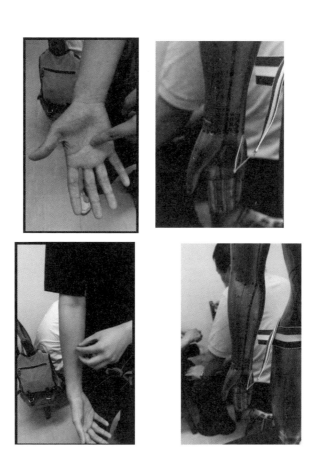

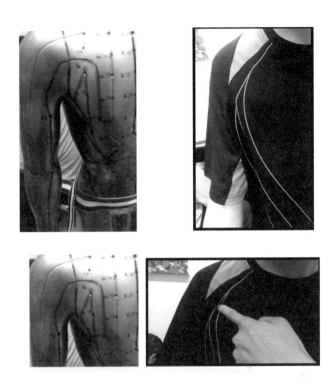

上圖: 透過病人皮膚觸痛點之描述，尋找相對應之經絡，例
如:心包經

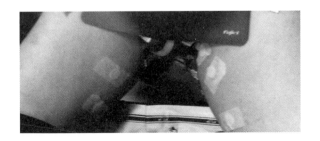

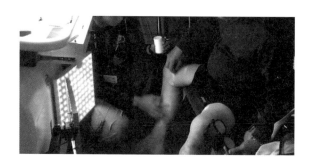

上圖: 把能量片貼合在經絡路線上，進行光照

(2)循經感傳（propagated sensation along meridians-PSM）現象

循經感傳是指針刺、生物能共振及其它方法刺激穴位時，人體出現一種酸、脹、麻等特殊感覺從受刺激的穴位開始，沿古典醫籍記載的經脈循行路線傳導的現象。

據中國的統計，發現循經感傳的出現率甚至觀察到，在 1000 人中有 7 人十二經絡都有顯著的循經感傳現象。通過對循經感傳現象和循經皮膚病的研究，學術界肯定了經絡現像是客觀存在的。

循經感傳（PSM）是一種沿經絡穴位的刺激的感傳移動。為了解釋經絡通道的真實結構，提出了一種"神經假說"。當針灸的穴位，通過感覺神經將信號提供給大腦，基本上，位置傳送刺激和經絡路線包圍含有運動

和感覺纖維神經束，而產生感覺。然而，傳播速度不像神經衝動的速度，而是慢慢感覺傳輸（例如，所記錄的速度約為 2-5 厘米/秒）。不管如何，透過循經感傳現象，同樣可以對照出可能經絡路線圖來找出病人需要治療的經絡，之後就可以把能量片貼合在經絡路線上，進行光照。

(3)經絡診斷及典型症狀

經絡	相關症狀
脾經	脾胃病，婦科，前陰病及經脈循行部位的其他病證。如胃脘痛、食則嘔、噯氣、腹脹、便溏、黃疸、身重無力、舌根強痛、下肢內側腫脹、厥冷、足大趾運動障礙；
胃經	胃腸病、頭面五官病、目、鼻、口、齒痛、頭痛、神志病，熱病及經脈循行部位的其他病證。如腸鳴腹脹，水腫，胃痛，嘔吐或消穀善饑，口渴，咽喉腫痛，鼻衄，胸部及膝臏等本經循行部位疼痛，皮膚病，口眼喎斜、高熱、汗出，發狂；
膽經	肝膽病，側頭、目、耳、咽喉病、胸脅病，神志病，熱病以及經脈循行部位的其他病

經絡	相關症狀
	證。如往來寒熱、口苦，目眩、視物不清，瘧疾，頭痛（偏頭痛），頷痛，目外眥痛，缺盆部腫痛，腋下腫，胸、脅、股、膝及下肢外側痛，足外側痛，足外側發熱，第四足趾處疼痛或運動障礙；
肝經	肝、膽、脾、胃病，婦科病，少腹、前陰病，以及經脈循行經過部位的其他病症。如腰痛，脅肋脹痛、胸悶，胸滿，呃逆、嘔吐、瀉泄、巔頂痛，遺尿，小便不利，疝氣，少腹腫痛、腰痛、月經不調、精神失常；
小腸經	頭面五官病（頭、項、耳、目、咽喉病），熱病，神志病以及經脈循行部位的其他病證。如少腹痛、腹脹、尿頻，腰脊痛引睪丸，耳聾，目黃，頰腫，咽喉腫痛、下頷及頸部疼痛，肩臂外側後緣痛；
心經	心、胸、神志病以及經脈循行部位的其他病證。如心痛，心前區疼痛、胸痛、出汗、心悸、失眠、咽干，口渴，目黃，脅痛，上臂內側痛（屈側後緣），厥冷，手心發熱；
大腸經	頭面五官疾患、熱病、皮膚病、腸胃病、神

經絡	相關症狀
	志病等及經脈循行部位的其他病症。如下牙痛、咽喉腫痛、鼻衄、鼻流清涕、口干、頸腫痛、上肢伸側前緣及肩部疼痛或運動障礙;
肺經	喉、胸、肺病,以及經脈循行部位的其他病證。如咳嗽,氣喘,少氣不足以息,咳血,傷風,胸部脹滿,咽喉腫痛,缺盆部及手臂內側前緣痛,肩背寒冷、疼痛;
膀胱經	頭面五官病、項、背、腰、下肢部病證以及神志病,背部第一側線的背俞穴及第二側線相平的腧穴,與其相關的臟腑病證和有關的組織器官病證。如小便不通,遺尿,癲狂,瘧疾,目痛,迎風流淚,鼻塞多涕,鼻衄,頭痛,項強、背腰臀部以及下肢後側本經循行部位疼痛;
腎經	婦科,前陰病,腎臟病,以及與腎有關的肺、心、肝、腦病,咽喉、舌等經脈循行經過部位的其他病症。如咳血,氣喘、咳嗽、頭昏目眩、舌干,咽喉腫痛,水腫、尿頻、遺尿、遺精、陽痿、小便不利、大便秘結或泄瀉、月經不調、腰痛,脊或股內後側痛,

經絡	相關症狀
	痿弱無力、下肢無力，足心熱；
三焦經	頭（側頭）、耳、目、胸脅、頰、咽喉病，熱病以及經脈循行部位的其他病證。如腹脹，水腫，遺尿，小便不利，耳鳴，耳聾，咽喉腫痛，目赤腫痛、目外眥痛，頰腫，耳後、肩臂肘部外側疼痛；
心包經	心、心包、胸、胃、神志病以及經脈循行部位的其他病證。如心痛、心前區痛，胸悶，心悸，心煩，癲狂、精神失常，腋腫，肘臂攣急、掌心發熱；

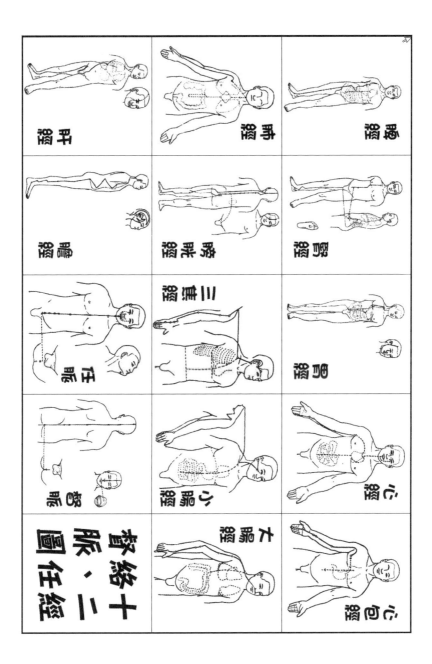

經肝　經肺　經胃

經膽　經胱膀　經腎

三焦經

任脈　經胃小　經心

腎脈　大腸經　心包經

十二經脈・絡脈圓住經

(4) 綜合以下：透過選擇 "觸發點"， "循經
感傳" 的現象或中國傳統醫學有關經絡診斷
及典型症狀

　　按照　"觸發點" 和 "循經感傳" 的現象等等方
式，所選擇的經絡通道上之穴位點，我們利用生物能量
貼片，置放在不正常穴位點所構成的經絡通道上，進行
生物光能共振照射，持續至少 15 分鐘，並進行每天兩
次照射共振。

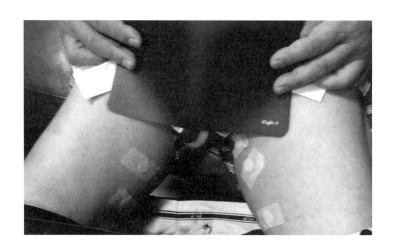

圖 2 操作

＜生物能產品使用須知＞

　　若使用生物能相關產品時產生頭暈，此為本材料正在調整體質加速血液循環為正常反應，請繼續使用短時間此現象將自然消失，若身體感覺酸痛乃為本材料加速體內新陳代謝之反應，此為能量適應中的現象，繼續使用，等待恢復體力 ，本系列產品小孩是可以放心使用的。孕婦要由醫師說明下使用。

生物光能色彩醫學

生物光能臨床應用

色彩光療

　　彩光療法的基本原理在於利用波能傳送細胞訊息。長久以來，自然醫療界人士體會到，只要精準地投入極細微刺激色彩，就可以引發最大的功效。

　　色彩作用於有機體上最著名且顯而易見的效果，由約翰歐特博士的影片「控索光譜」中呈現過，利用顯微鏡觀察水蘊草細胞內葉綠粒（其細胞成分包含葉綠素）的活動模式，歐特博士發現，在自然的陽光下，所有葉綠粒都按照典型的水流模式，在細胞內有秩序圍繞著移動，然而，若將光線中過濾掉「紫」外線，許多葉綠粒即失去原有流向，而在細胞內會呈現行動遲緩的一團葉綠粒。歐特博士進一步的研究發現，大自然中細胞的改變似乎和人類的行為模式相近，行為會讓有些人習慣處於某特定模式，有些則放棄這個模式，而有些簡化或放棄對環境、或對特殊光譜部份。隨著人們類大多數時間缺少陽光的均衡滋養，使得有些行為和生理機能產生差異，舉例來說，習慣性戴太陽眼鏡或持續在人工照明系統下可能導致如同吃不均衡的飲食容易營不良。自從一

八○○年（十九世紀）全球的醫生留意到光的治療特質，此時，稱「光」利用在症狀的治療上，從單純的發炎、麻痺、癱瘓到結核病，接著開始注意光的顏色及彩虹光的效果。賈寇柏.賴勃曼博士發現使用太陽的熱光和電子藍光組合來刺激人體的腺體，一般為神經系統和分泌器官，有特殊且特別的效能。因此，「光」成了治療疾病的主要元素，尤其是對已轉變成慢性病，或內分泌系統、腺體機能失調引發的症狀，「光」可使之重現生機，回復秩序。

（引用自賈寇柏.賴勃曼博士的—「光，未來的醫學一書」）

人類早期應用陽光施行彩光療法，因為太陽光包含完整光譜色彩。生物需要陽光才能生存，太陽光能源產生所有顏色的波長，從紫外線、可見光到紅外線大略均勻的分布，這就是所知道的完整光譜的白色光。普通的人工照明無法放射出像自然光一般平衡的色彩，因為在某些波長的光會高過於其他的光。俄羅斯的臨床與實驗醫學研究中心在臨床經驗中發現，運用在身體的光，視顏色的頻率而定，會穿透身體 0.2 到 0.3 公分深；科學家發現身體只有某些特定的部位能在表層之下轉換光，而這些部位則和針灸穴點相對應；重要的是他們發現光在身體中是透過經絡網在指揮運作的，這一點正與古印度和中國文化所發現的能量通道相符合。

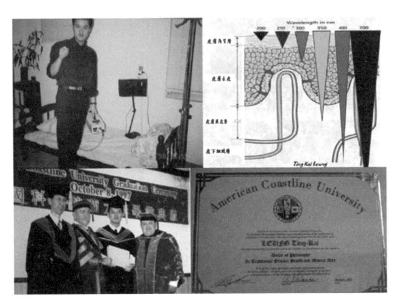

1997 年 10 月獲美國科斯蘭大學頒發東方醫學博士學位

　　以「氦—氖」可見紅光（632.8 奈米波長）雷射
（red helium-neon laser light: 632.8nm）為主題發表了以
可見光光能於各病例上的臨床應用研究論文，獲頒發博
士學位

　　1998 年攝於臨床工作，研究的主題:「氦－氖」可
見紅光（632.8 奈米波長）雷射（red helium-neon laser
light: 632.8nm）（圖中手上所提的設備），發表了以可
見光光能於各病例上之臨床應用研究論文，背後病床上
的是自行組合的特定彩色光譜燈源。

生物光能的發展

　　生物光能是建基於生物陶瓷能的特性，加上使用可見光光譜的波長（390 至 750nm），行成紅外光光譜內的"光激發光"效應，強化前面提到生物陶瓷能所原本產生之物理，生物和物理化學作用，然後傳遞到遠距離或滲透組織的深層。

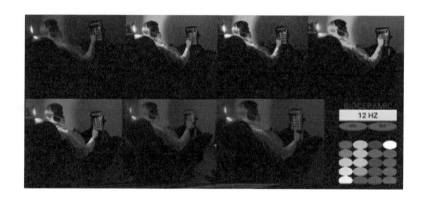

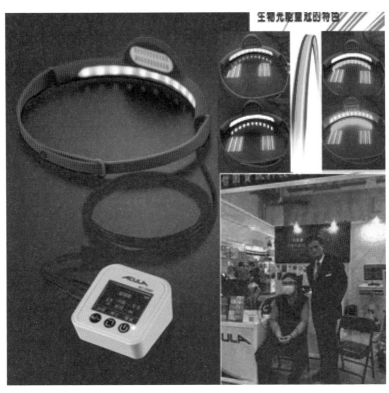

已經証明次生物光廳色彩臨床效果

<色彩生物光能的作用參考>

色彩生物光能—顏色	產生之感受	建議
紅	某處骨骼肌肉關節有感/變強(5)；心跳加速(1)；喉嚨有東西感(1)；打嗝(1)；熱感/內熱()；煩悶(1)；刺激皮	皮膚瘙癢者不建議使用 建議使用在

色彩生物光能—顏色	產生之感受	建議
	膚的微循環(1)；頭頂脹(2)；眼部有脹感(2)；刺激皮膚瘙癢；全身流動感(1)；做完精神好(1)；口腔痛惑(1)	元氣不足者
橙	幫助睡眠(2)某處疼痛(4)；心跳加速(1)；刺激微循環(1)	
黃	腸子滾動(3)；打嗝(2)；某處疼痛(1)；呼吸沈重(1)；背部有感(1)；身體搖晃/旋轉(1)；心情愉快(1)；舒服感(1)	調整腸胃
綠	幫助睡眠(10)；舒服感(2)；腸子滾動(1)；身體遙晃感(1)；耳部有聲音；背部有感(2)；能量流動(1)；不明流動感強烈(2)；看到閃光(1)；頭頂脹(1)	失眠，焦慮，緊張者失建議使用
藍	腸道排氣(1)；頭部有感(1)；喉嚨有東西感(1)；呼吸沈重(1)；足底有感(2)；全身流動感(1)；幫助睡眠(1)	
綻	鼻子有感(1)；喉嚨有東西感(2)；眼睛有感(1)；頭頂脹感(2)；心跳加速(1)；某處骨骼肌肉關節有感(1)；呼吸沈重(1)；緊張後想睡(1)	
紫	感受輕鬆(4)；之後變精神(2)；幫助	(1) 考慮使

166

色彩生物光能—顏色	產生之感受	建議
	睡眠(2)；心跳加速(2)；頭腦變清楚(1)；緩解頭痛(1)；記憶力加強(1)；身體搖晃/旋轉(1)；全身流動感(1)；某處骨骼肌肉關節有感(1)；左腦痛感(1)；發汗(1)	用在加強腦部功能(2)失眠，焦慮，緊張者建議使用

生物能虛擬現實意識科技(BIO VR Relax)
—針對身心症狀和情緒問題

(1)人的情緒問題

　　醫學研究顯示，人對不良情緒忍耐克制，或者鬱悶壓抑時，會對身心健康帶來重大傷害。本研究是建基於「光聲激發生物能量材（BIOCERAMIC）—生物光能共振」技術，已經臨床使用後，發現對於情緒改善有顯著效果。在之前的研究成果，亦曾利用功能磁振造影（fMRI）和給予「生物光能共振」技術，比較治療前和治療後，對於心理性睡眠障礙患者除症狀有所改善，同時結果發現相應的大腦和小腦區域的激發現象，和文獻上一上精神情緒性疾病有相關性。

　　近年來，台灣人情緒問題，包括憂鬱和煩燥情緒的問題盛行率有逐漸增加的趨勢，青少年情緒問題不僅影響患者身心健康、人際關係及學業表現，也經常造成家庭與學校照顧上沈重的負擔，進而耗費相當大的社會成本。因而，快樂（Happiness）的研究越來越受到重視。

　　部分的青少年憂鬱情緒是以易怒與叛逆來呈現，如果忽略這些已出現的憂鬱情緒，常導致無法早期發現、早期治療，進而造成許多不良的惡性後果，如藥物濫

用、行為問題、自我傷害、或自殺，以至於被注意時都已為時太晚。若能藉由有效的篩檢工具發現這些高危險群，及時介入處理，則可避免不必要的遺憾。

隨著情感計算和智慧化的人機交互介面的發展,發展具備感知和理解人的情感的能力。其中，面部表情分析是一個較直接和重要的課題被提出來，並在近十多年來展開了廣泛的研究。目前已有多種面部表情識別方法,但是對表情強度的度量並沒有充分展開。對面部表情進行強度度量有助於進一步理解人的情感狀態和情緒強度,是情感機器人的未來發展趨勢。

(2)虛擬現實催眠（VR Hypnosis）

過去二十年，催眠作為治療疼痛的有效性能力的科學證據已經普及，然而它的廣泛使用已經受到諸如臨床醫生的支持。

但傳統催眠作為治療受限於專業治療師技術，時間和精力等有限因素, 無法隨時提供催眠治療，以及患者對催眠放鬆是否有效之認知。

開發虛擬現實催眠（VR Hypnosis）的理論是應用三維的，身臨其境的，虛擬的現實技術來引導患者通過傳統催眠放鬆時所使用類似的步驟。虛擬現實取代了許多患者在傳統催眠放鬆必須主動努力用想像才能幻想出來的刺激, 這種刺激一般是要通過催眠治療師的口頭提

示（suggestion）才可以想像出來。虛擬現實意識科技（VR Relax）的目的是探討如何虛擬現實可能有助於提供沒有催眠治療師下，產生類似催眠放鬆之效果。

　　針對一些情緒緊張、無法放鬆和長期失眠之患者，在使用「生物光能共振」技術時，觀察到「生物光能共振」能強化原來正念放鬆（mindfulness）之效果。但是如果要所有對像都接受「生物光能共振」之對象都自己執行正念放鬆（mindfulness）比較困難。於是，我們初步開發出「生物光能共振」專用的虛擬現實意識科技（VR Relax）的影音視聽系統。VR 是利用電腦技術模擬出一個立體、高解釋度的 3D 空間，當使用者穿戴特殊顯示裝置，會產生身處現實一般的錯覺，產生身歷其境、甚至有刺激感和愉悅感。VR 有很多應用，不只用在遊戲，亦可以應用在緩和情緒問題和腦神經退化身心疾病也可以派上用場，像是在醫學上方面研究出臨床測試出可以改善藥物濫用、焦慮和抑鬱症等症狀。

　　一直以來，心理疾病是一個殺人於無形的兇手，近年更呈現年輕化的趨勢。但隨著科技進步，VR Relax 也許能成為這個問題的解決方案之一，從「生物光能共振」切入，合併成為一套整合的系統（BIORelax VR），其使用將改善人的心理健康問題。在 BIORelax VR 的基礎下，我們將進一步開發虛擬現實—身心語言程式學（VR-NLP），身心語言程式學，即 Neuro-

Linguistic Programming（簡稱 NLP）。NLP 是一種治療技術，用於檢測和重新規劃無意識的思想和行為模式，以改變心理反應。NLP 發展自美國加州大學聖塔克魯茲（Santa Cruz）分校，發展者聲稱，神經過程（神經），語言和通過經驗（編程）學習的行為模式之間存在聯繫，因此它可以用於教育和醫學領域如有放於恐懼症，焦慮和抑鬱症。NLP 是一個多層次的學習過程，通常包括建立醫生和患者之間的關係，收集心理內在信息和健康期望的結果定義（desired health outcome definition），以及使用諸如問題集等技術（sets of questions）和工具以促進患者思維和行為的改變。NLP 技術一般需要專人引導，接受者亦必須主動努力用想像才能幻想出指定的思考刺激，這種刺激一般是要通過 NLP 治療師的口頭提示（human oral suggestions）才可以想像出來。在本研究中，我們將進一步招攬軟體工程師，協助開發虛擬現實—身心語言程式學（VR-NLP）的自動化平台模板。簡單來說，先透過 BIORelax VR 系統來引導患者達到放鬆，虛擬現實意識科技（VR Relax）之目的是利用 BIORelax VR 運作下，以軟體程式產生合適使用對象的心理情緒問題所需要的自動（人功智能）語言提示（artificial suggestions）來取代人功的口頭提示（human oral suggestions），收集心理內在信息和提升健康期望，最終達到改變不當行為模式，改

變問題認知和改善心理情緒問題。另外，針對腦神經退化人仕，我們亦會在「生物光能共振」運作下，先產生腦部微循環和相關刺激，另外軟體工程師將設計和提供不同的身歷其境、刺激感和愉悅感的 VR 影音程式，透過專業評估，來了解是否能改善腦神經退化之症狀。

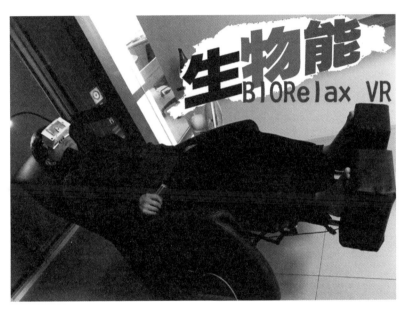

本研究為合併「生物光能共振」和虛擬現實意識科技（VR Relax）核評估 其對身心症狀和情緒問題之效果

生物能量意識—21 世紀「元宇宙」保健養生應用

　　「生物能元宇宙」是建築在「生物光能共振」第五力場所產生對人類意識提升現象的基礎上，而另外發展生物能虛擬實境平台-----仲屏號意識系統。首先，要先解釋何為「意識」，一般來說，腦（brain）、意識（consciousness）、思想（mind）應該連在一起看。腦、意識是範圍比較小的層次，更高的層次是思想。在討論意識的時候，醫學界通常認為有兩種，一種是廣義的意識，包括自我意識，談的是主觀性的東西，它和精神醫學、心理學有關；另一種是狹義的意識，談的是客觀的東西，和腦神經生理學有關。根據瑞士心理學家榮格（C.G.Jung）論述，一個人之人格組成成份包括：意識、個人潛意識和集體潛意識。而「生物能元宇宙」保健技術是要創造一個「身心靈」的情境來串通意識和潛意識，意圖啟發人類潛能和自我療癒機制。

以下介紹「生物能元宇宙」-- 仲屏號意識影音系統包含之內容：

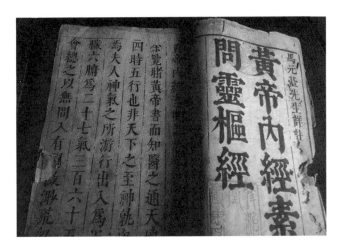

整合東方經絡學說

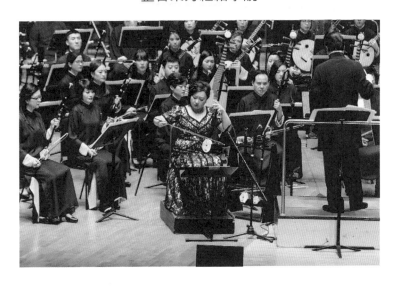

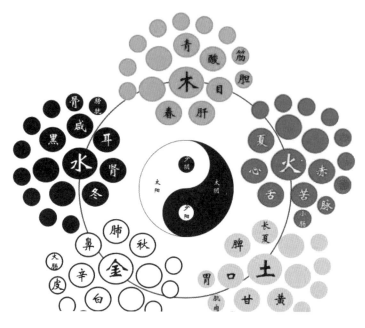

五行影音

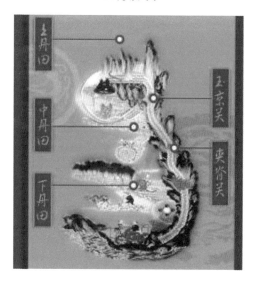

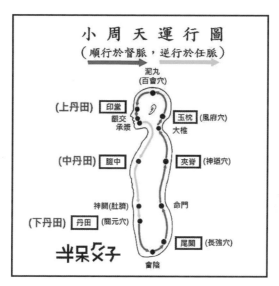

道學內丹

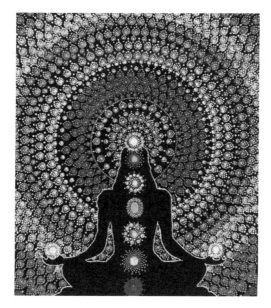

印度脈輪

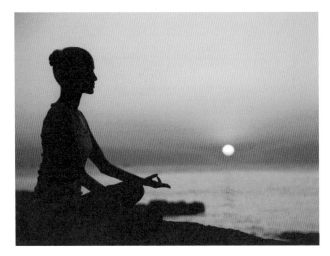

正念冥想

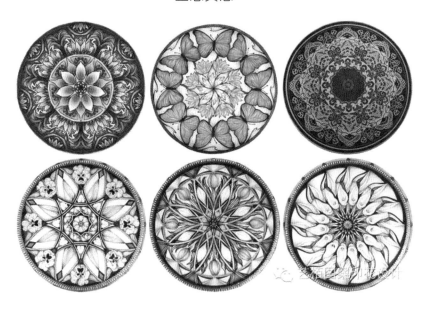

神聖幾何 /動態曼陀羅

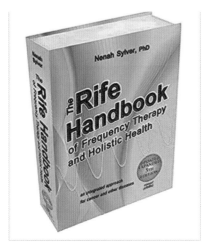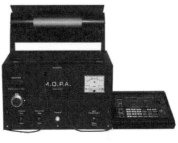

高頻波平衡頻率自然調理法　(Rife/Spooky Frequency)

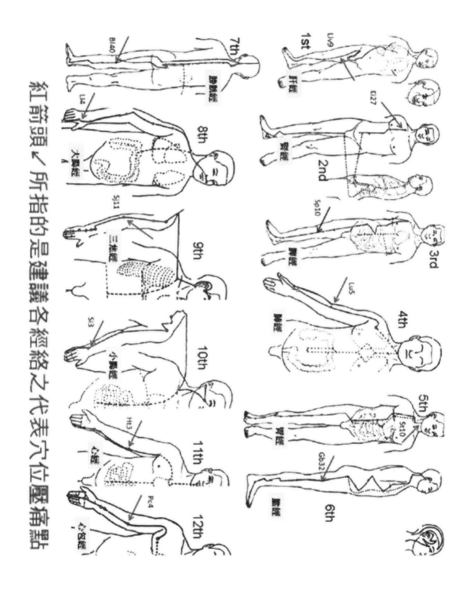

紅箭頭/所指的是建議各經絡之代表穴位壓痛點

心臟十二諧波音節拍共振缺氧壓痛記錄表

心臟十二諧波音節拍	作用前疼痛分數	作用後疼痛分數
第一諧波音節拍 肝經(LIV9)		
第二諧波音節拍 腎經(K27)		
第三諧波音節拍 脾經(SP10)		
第四諧波音節拍 肺經(LU5)		
第五諧波音節拍 胃經(St10)		
第六諧波音節拍 膽經(Gb32)		
第七諧波音節拍 膀胱經(Bl40)		
第八諧波音節拍 大腸(Li4)		
第九諧波音節拍 三焦(Sj11)		
第十諧波音節拍 小腸(Si3)		
第十一諧波音節拍 心經(Ht3)		
第十二諧波音節拍 心包(Pc4)		

不痛　　一點點痛　　輕微痛　　很痛　　非常痛　　無法忍受的痛

0　1　2　3　4　5　6　7　8　9　10

彩色生物能應用原則

- 生物綠色放鬆和睡眠
- 生物紅色肌肉和低血壓;虛弱;長期關節病;
- 生物藍光是能量急性痛/鎮定劑
- 生物紫色啟動腦細胞；有利腦神經退化
- 生物黃色胃腸道系統問題
- 生物橙光針對月經痛,憂鬱症,寒冷
- 生物淺藍光是針對喉嚨/甲狀腺

生物色彩光能調理，按中醫基礎理論

生物能色彩光	中醫屬性	功能
藍色	(水)為純陰	(寒,用於陰虛火旺)
紅色	(火)為純陽	(熱,用於陽虛火衰)
綠色(黃加藍)	為抑木(肝亢)扶土(脾虛)	是安定平衡之光(用在肝實証加失眠)
黃(橘)色	(屬土)為陽中之陰	扶脾陽養胃陰,平衡脾胃功能之光
紫(靛)色(藍加紅)	為陰中之陽	陰陽並補,益精填髓,入腦,屬清明之光

生物光能貼片與軟體系統使用說明

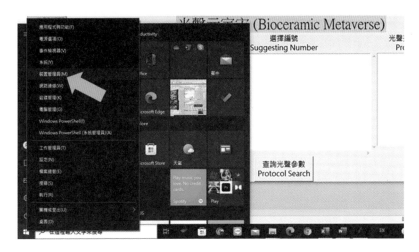

點選裝置管理員(M)

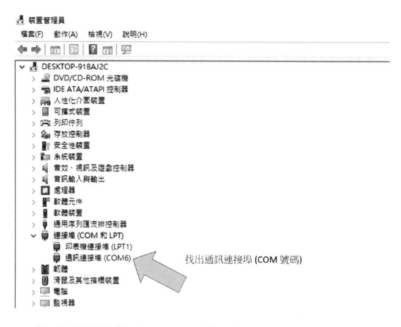

找出通訊連接埠 (COM 號碼)

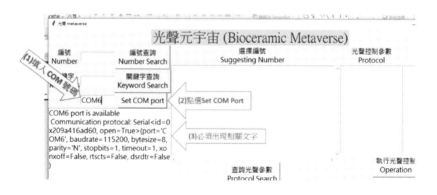

填入 COM 號碼/Set COM Port/

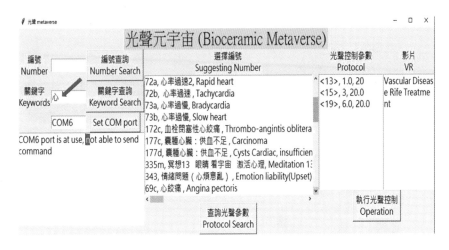

仲屏號生物能系統之關鍵字查詢, 配對出最合適療
癒的光聲控制參數和 VR 影片

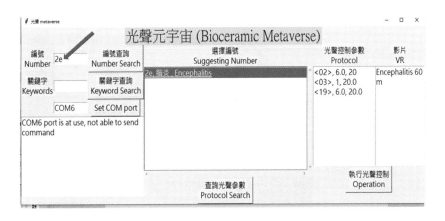

仲屏號生物能系統之編號查詢, 配對出最合適療癒
的光聲控制參數和 VR 影片

<生物光能共振人功智能化：元宇宙遠距保健建設工程>

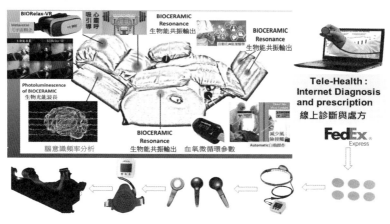

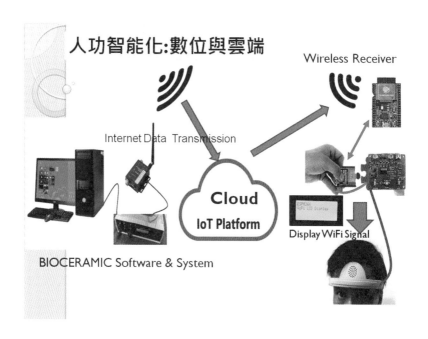

＜生物能軟體系統(光能貼片) 應用說明＞
本軟體為生物光能專用

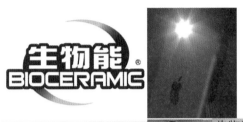

生物能量貼片
主成份：
純天然植物生物能量
榮獲台灣、大陸、日本、美國、德國發明專利

生物能e學院

步驟一：

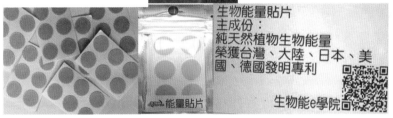

關鍵字查詢 ←--- 任選其中之一 ---→ 編號查詢

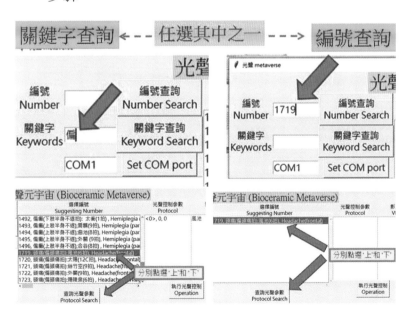

186

步驟二：

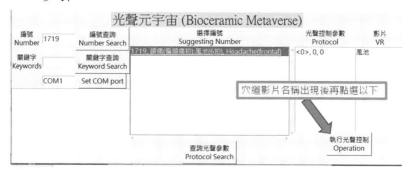

步驟三：

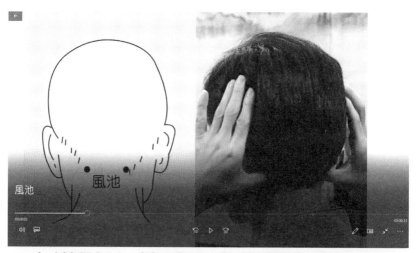

•穴道影片:協助取穴位置自動放影

187

＜生物能網站應用說明＞

https://www.bioceraenergy.com/knowledge/

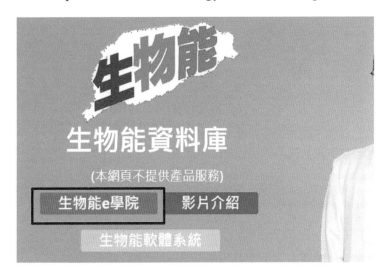

http://www.bioceraenergy.com/bioceramic_system/

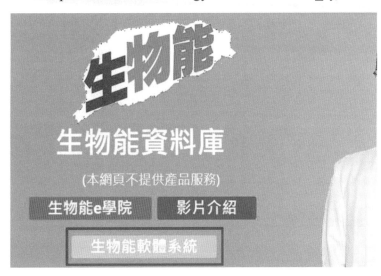

生物能再生醫學

經絡再生醫學概念

首先，人類心跳每分鐘僅消耗約 1.3 瓦的能量，消耗傳統燈泡五十分之一電力,能驅動全身超過十二萬公里的血管網絡，維持血液循環。這是因為每次心跳產生的諧波頻率，在器官和微血管中形成特定的共振模式。根據研究，這些頻率對應人體主要器官，例如：如果基礎心跳頻率為一分鐘 72 次 即其基礎心跳為 1.2 Hz

心跳會產生「十一」加「一」諧波頻率的多重諧波頻率，與中醫十二經絡的傳播路線是相符的。

諧波音節拍 (Harmonic Sound Beat)	經絡名稱 (Meridian Name)	代表點穴位 (Representative Acupoint)
第一諧波音節拍	肝經 (Liver Meridian)	陰包　LV9
第二諧波音節拍	腎經 (Kidney Meridian)	腧府　K27
第三諧波音節拍	脾經 (Spleen Meridian)	血海　SP10

第四諧波音節拍	肺經 (Lung Meridian)	尺澤 LU5
第五諧波音節拍	胃經 (Stomach Meridian)	水突 ST10
第六諧波音節拍	膽經 (Gallbladder Meridian)	風市 GB32
第七諧波音節拍	膀胱經 (Bladder Meridian)	委中 BL40
第八諧波音節拍	大腸經 (Large Intestine Meridian)	合谷 LI4
第九諧波音節拍	三焦 (Triple Burner Meridian)	清冷淵 SJ11
第十諧波音節拍	小腸 (Small Intestine Meridian)	腕骨 SI3
第十一諧波音節拍	心經 (Heart Meridian)	少海 HT3
第十二諧波音節拍	心包經 (Pericardium Meridian)	曲澤 PC4

　　每個器官對應特定的諧波頻率，形成共振效應，促進微血管的血液灌流注到各別器官。諧波頻率增強微血管中的血流動性，支持細胞代謝及組織修復。

有關穴位與經絡的科學意義

穴位就是諧波頻率通道(中醫講的經絡)路線上所對應的波動路線能量集中點，同時亦是感覺神經集中點。經絡網絡被認為是全身共振通道，功能是減少心臟負擔,促進微循環,促進血液組織器官微灌流 perfusion。提供心跳的低耗能環境、卻能維持高效率循環系統藉由心跳諧波頻率傳遞能量，協助器官功能與疾病調理，能激發細胞活性和促進組織修復。

再生醫學

再生醫學是一門致力於修復或再生人體受損組織和器官的醫學領域。在自然界中，某些動物如壁虎等，當牠們面臨危險時，會脫落部分身體，例如尾巴或肢體，並能夠再生出新的部分。再生醫學就是類似透過研究這些動物的再生能力，尋找方法促進人類自身組織的修復和再生，以治療各種疾病和創傷。

生物陶瓷能技術在傳統中醫經絡理論中扮演的角色

簡單來說，生物陶瓷能的研究與開發旨在創造一種能量，該能量能夠與人體心跳產生的諧波音頻頻率共同

傳導（類似於選擇性地在不同捷運路線上行駛），從而促進不同經絡通道的血液微循環，並具備生物效應和再生醫學的概念。具體而言，生物陶瓷能技術的聲波振動與光能刺激執行模式具有以下優點：

1. **非侵入性**：不同於傳統中醫的針灸療法，生物陶瓷能光聲體外刺激技術不需要通過針刺穿透皮膚進入體內，避免了侵入性操作帶來的不舒服和風險。

2. **物理作用**：該技術通過物理學的方法作用於人體，無需口服藥物，減少了藥物攝入可能引發的風險，同時降低了由於中藥品質參差不齊、農藥殘留或其他污染問題所帶來的副作用，提供了一種更為安全和自然的治療方式。

3. **多重能量供應**：生物陶瓷能不僅利用聲波的諧音共振來促進氣血流通，還結合了安全的可見光波長生物能技術，為人體提供多層次的能量支持。這些技術結合了傳統中醫的補益、中和和清熱等內在能量調節概念，通過現代科技手段，實現對人體內在能量的全面調理與平衡。

此外，生物陶瓷能技術的數位化特性使其能夠根據不同的經絡道選擇相應的頻率參數，這有利於 AI 人工智能和網路雲端控制等數位科技的發展。這種技術幫助將過去抽象的傳統醫學理念公開化、具體化，儀器化，

並與現代醫學同步發展，打造一個物理醫學平台。

通過這些特性，生物陶瓷能技術能夠有效促進經絡系統的氣血流通，提升整體健康水平，並支持再生醫學的發展。這種技術將現代生物工程與傳統中醫理論有機結合，不僅為疾病治療提供創新手段，也為健康管理帶來更全面和高效的解決方案。

生物陶瓷技術如何幫助西方主流醫學家和基礎醫學家理解傳統中醫（特別是經絡系統）

生物陶瓷技術的有效性和可重複性，不僅證明了傳統中醫理論的真實性，還為西方醫學理解中醫經絡系統提供了科學依據，具體體現在以下幾個方面：

1. 經絡的科學基礎：

   駐波現象：心跳產生的諧波頻率形成了「駐波」，生物陶瓷技術支持經絡系統是由這些駐波形成的。在動脈和微循環系統中，這些駐波產生固定的節點和反節點，對應中醫的穴位位置，提供了經絡傳導現象的現代物理解釋。

2. 微循環與氣血運行的關聯：

   生物陶瓷技術增強微循環，促進細胞間液體和微血管中血液的流動，模擬中醫「氣血運行」的概念，驗證了經絡作為氣血傳導通道的功能

性存在。

3. **頻率與器官共振的支持：**

根據心跳的諧波頻率，每個內臟器官對應特定的共振頻率。生物陶瓷技術模擬並放大這些共振效應，幫助理解中醫「臟腑功能」和「經絡調節」的生理基礎。

4. **穴位的能量集中點**

人體共有 365 個穴位，與一年 365 天相呼應；人體的 12 條經絡也與一年 12 個月相對應。在西方主流醫學中，骨科和復健科醫師經常遇到病患的身體疼痛點，通常被稱為「肌筋膜疼痛發炎」。根據復健科學期刊的研究，這些疼痛點通常是由微循環問題導致的，例如肌肉緊繃、缺血、缺氧。生物陶瓷技術通過短時間的作用，即可有效緩解這些疼痛。我們的多篇研究論文證實，這並非單點的問題，而是一個整體通道的問題。當微循環恢復正常後，這些疼痛點便能迅速改善。這些研究進一步驗證了生物陶瓷技術所揭示的經絡諧波、音共振與微循環的真實性及其科學客觀存在，為中醫經絡理論提供了堅實的現代化科學基礎。

5. **跨學科融合：**

⊙結合材料科學、生物物理學和分子生物學，

生物陶瓷技術為中醫經絡提供了量化的研究模型。通過大數據和 AI 雲端計算分析，使中醫理論進一步數據化，促進了中醫與主流醫學的學術合作。

6.替代與輔助治療應用：

⊙生物陶瓷技術作為經絡系統的非侵入性替代方案，能顯著改善睡眠障礙、疼痛和炎症，有助於減少化學藥物的使用，降低藥物副作用和依賴風險。

結論：

生物陶瓷技術將物理學、心血管生理學與中醫概念相結合，為經絡和其他中醫理論提供了科學化的解釋。不僅加深了西方醫學對中醫的理解，還為中醫教育和技術傳承提供了現代化的基礎。

目前在生物陶瓷能再生醫學實際的應用有哪些？哪些疾病（族群）可以因此受惠？

生物陶瓷能技術再生醫學的臨床有效性與傳統中醫經絡治療類似，其核心不僅針對某一特定疾病，而是針對患者的整體狀況進行全面分析和分類。主要概念是先將各種疾病的不適感，包括心理和生理層面，歸納到特

定的經絡共振頻率問題上。同時，根據患者內在能量狀態，判斷其需求是補充能量、平衡調和，還是清熱排毒，從而實現精準的能量調理和治療對應。

根據我們多年的經驗，疾病在急性期（從幾個小時到三週內）通常伴隨著較嚴重的發炎反應，而這種急性發炎期往往會壓迫或影響到某一條經絡。此時，針對清熱的光波長以及對應的經絡共振頻率治療，可以有效緩解疼痛指數。此外，結合適當的藥物治療，效果通常會更加顯著。

在經絡處於急性狀態時，我們一再強調要儘快緩解病理性發炎狀態，這段關鍵時期約為三週到三個月。此期間應使用對應的物理方法，以防止病情進一步發展為慢性狀態。

一旦相關疾病進入慢性階段（持續三個月以上），通常會出現各種症狀和能量問題。此時，治療需要更大的耐心，這個時間生物能量共振配合內在體質能量補益會是這個時間較常用的方法，並結合長期、固定、反覆使用的物理工具進行調理，最終目標是實現完全康復。

生物陶瓷能再生醫學的有效對範圍與適用族群

如上述所言，生物能共振再生醫學與能量醫學，或傳統中醫經絡相關的調理，主要以能量分類為原則，而非僅針對某一單一疾病，並同時在生理與心理層面進行

調整。

如果需要更具體了解我們已發表論文中涉及的相關疾病和案例資料，我們可以提供一份列表，將論文依序排序供大家參考。此外，也可以提供更具體的研究成果項目，以及所對應的發表論文編號，方便查閱。

以下是主要的應用範疇及其受益的疾病和族群（參見已發表論文內容）：

1.骨骼重建與修復

骨折治療：生物陶瓷材能照射，促進新骨形成，加速骨折癒合。

骨質疏鬆症：增強骨密度，預防骨折風險，提升生活品質。運動損傷康復：生物陶瓷技術促進肌肉和韌帶的修復，提高運動員的康復效率。

女性（70 歲）：結合生物陶瓷技術與幹細胞療法，顯著加速脊椎壓迫性骨折的癒合，3 個月後背痛減輕，能自行行走。

腦退化神經退行性疾病/帕金森氏症：生物陶瓷技術通過調節神經系統活動，促進神經再生，減緩病情進展。

神經損傷修復：促進神經纖維的再生，提高功能恢復效果。（參見第 16 篇）

中風後康復：生物陶瓷技術促進中風後神經功

能的恢復，提高患者的生活質量。（參見第 28 篇）

2.慢性病管理

高血壓與糖尿病：改善微循環，提升血液供應和氧氣輸送，有助於控制血壓和血糖水平，減少併發症風險。

心血管疾病：促進血管內皮修復，預防動脈硬化，保護心血管健康。

3.疼痛管理與炎症緩解

肌筋膜疼痛發炎：生物陶瓷技術通過改善微循環和減少肌肉緊繃，快速緩解慢性疼痛和炎症。（參見第 33 篇、34 篇）

慢性腰痛與關節炎：有效減輕疼痛，提升關節功能，改善生活品質。（參見第 13、17 篇）

成功案例：

男性（45 歲）：長期慢性腰痛患者，經過 8 周的生物陶瓷治療後，腰痛明顯減輕，活動度增加，基本無疼痛感。

4.心理壓力與睡眠障礙

失眠與焦慮：生物陶瓷技術調節自律神經系統，改善睡眠質量，緩解焦慮情緒。（參見第 31 篇、32 篇）

心理健康：減少壓力，提高情緒穩定性，提升

整體心理健康狀態。（參見第 35 篇、36 篇）

成功案例：

男性（45 歲）：長期失眠患者，接受 5 次生物陶瓷治療後，睡眠質量顯著改善，焦慮情緒緩解，工作效率提高。（參見第 13 篇）

5.運動損傷與康復

肌肉拉傷與韌帶扭傷：生物陶瓷技術促進組織修復，縮短康復時間，提高運動表現。（參見第 6 篇、15 篇）

運動員康復：提高運動員的恢復效率，預防運動傷病。（參見第 15 篇）

案例：

運動員康復：運動員在接受生物陶瓷治療後，運動表現和康復速度顯著提升，傷後復健效果更佳。（參見第 15 篇）

6.美容與皮膚護理

皮膚再生/傷口癒合：促進膠原蛋白合成，促進傷口癒合，減少疤痕形成。

受惠族群

老年人：特別是患有骨質疏鬆、慢性病和神經退行性疾病的高齡患者。

中青年人：在壓力管理、睡眠改善和運動損傷康復方面受益顯著。

運動員：用於運動損傷的預防和康復，提高運動表現和抗壓能力。

慢性病患者：如高血壓、糖尿病患者，通過生物陶瓷技術改善健康狀況。

美容與皮膚護理需求者：希望改善皮膚質量、促進傷口癒合和減少疤痕的患者。

7.普遍反應

普遍反應 1：長期失眠和焦慮，接受生物陶瓷治療後，睡眠質量顯著改善，情緒穩定性提高，工作效率也有所提升。

普遍反應 2：運動員在接受生物陶瓷刺激後，運動表現和康復速度顯著提升，能更快地重返賽場，並取得了更好的成績。

普遍反應 3：我們在中華科技大學長期進行的研究發現，無論是何種亞健康狀態的個案，只要接受過我們的生物能再生醫學服務，他們的情緒和心情普遍會變得愉悅，同時也顯著減少對精神藥物及安眠藥的依賴。

結論

根據相關研究論文，生物能再生醫學結合生物陶瓷技術已在骨骼修復、神經再生、慢性病管理、疼痛緩解、心理健康、運動康復和皮膚護理等多個醫學領域取

得了顯著成效。這些應用不僅提高了治療效果，還提升了患者的生活品質。

在生物陶瓷能再生醫學中，合併幹細胞再生技術是如何被應用？

從父母結合形成的受精卵開始，發展為最初的幹細胞，隨後逐漸分化為各種細胞組織。再生療法，例如幹細胞治療和外泌體療法等，正是基於再生醫學的核心理念，利用幹細胞的分化能力修復因疾病或老化而受損的細胞，恢復身體正常功能，為現代醫學帶來了重要突破。

同樣的原理在胚胎的物理發展：

人體經絡的物理通道，實際上是各種諧波頻率通道的具體表現。在器官和微血管中，這些通道形成了特定的共振模式，例如肝臟、腎臟、脾臟、肺部、胃部、膽經、膀胱、大腸、腹膜（三焦）、小腸、心臟和心包等主要器官。這些共振通道的設定，基於內在的邏輯與系統性關聯，展現了人體器官協同運作與調節的機制，其發展可追溯至胚胎階段。

有關 光與聲波對幹細胞的促進作用的相關國際論文發表

研究表明，不同波長的光和聲波頻率能積極影響幹細胞的增殖與分化：

可見光效應：

- **紅光**：促進骨分化，助於骨骼再生。
- **綠光**：加速幹細胞向神經細胞分化，激活相關信號通路。
- **藍光**：促進神經生成，有助於神經損傷修復。

振動與聲波刺激的幹細胞研究成果

振動促進骨分化：提升膠原蛋白生成，

聲波增強多能性：促進人類胚胎幹細胞增殖與功能性。

聲波對高齡幹細胞優化：改善高齡患者脂肪幹細胞的骨分化能力。

聲波微環境調節：優化骨髓間充質幹細胞生成骨與軟骨的微環境。

臨床應用與未來展望

1.**實際應用體**

骨再生與骨質疏鬆：非侵入性骨損傷修復，加速骨

重建。

神經退化疾病：延緩神經退化，改善功能。

心理與睡眠改善：調節自律神經，緩解炎症，提高睡眠質量。

慢性病管理：精準頻率治療，適用於個性化醫療需求。

2.未來展望

隨著臨床研究的深入，生物陶瓷技術結合光與聲學刺激，為骨關節、神經修復及慢性病治療領域提供創新突破。透過精準的頻率應用，該技術將成為幹細胞外泌再生醫學的重要輔助工具，進一步提升醫療效果與患者生活品質。

生物能皇冠經絡數字

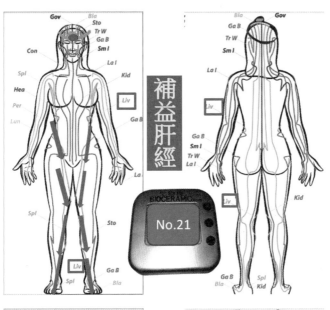

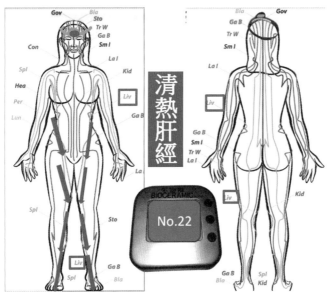

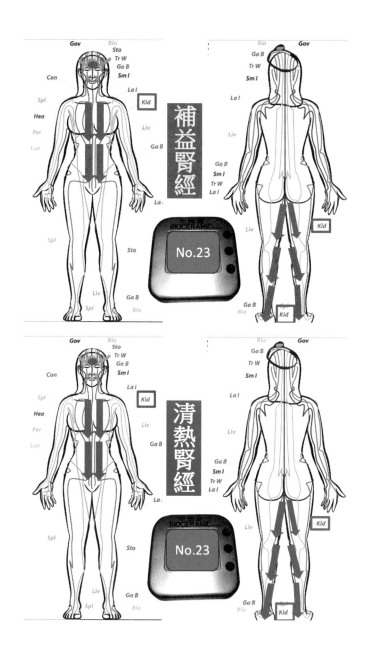

補益腎經

清熱腎經

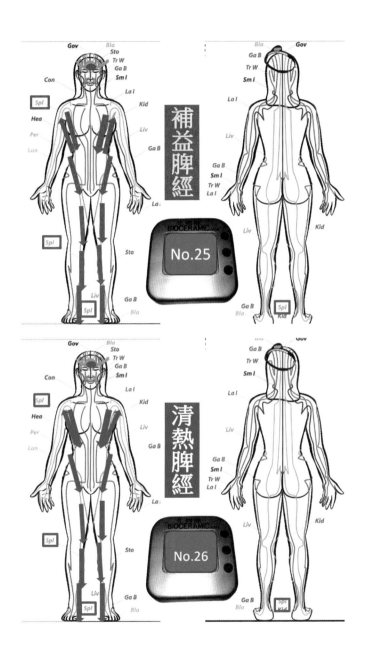

補益脾經

No.25

清熱脾經

No.26

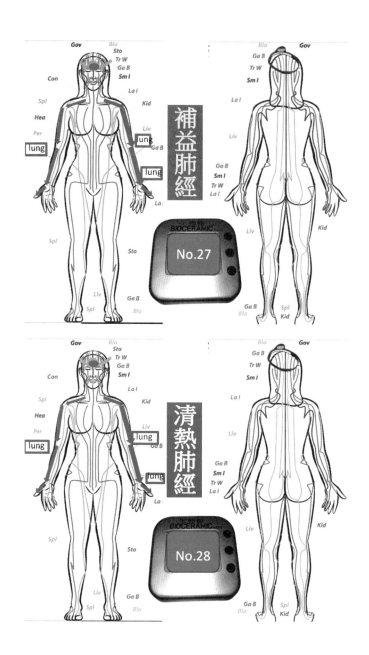

補益肺經

No.27

清熱肺經

No.28

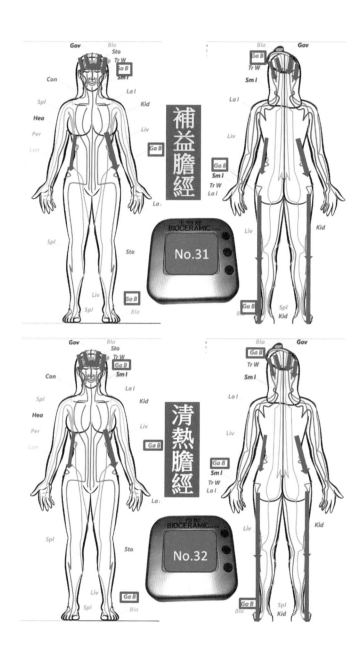

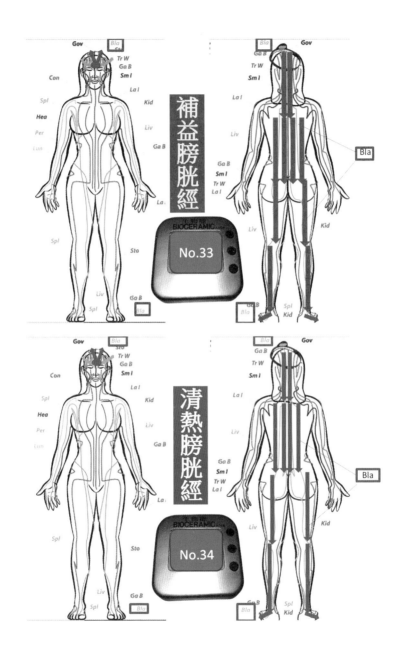

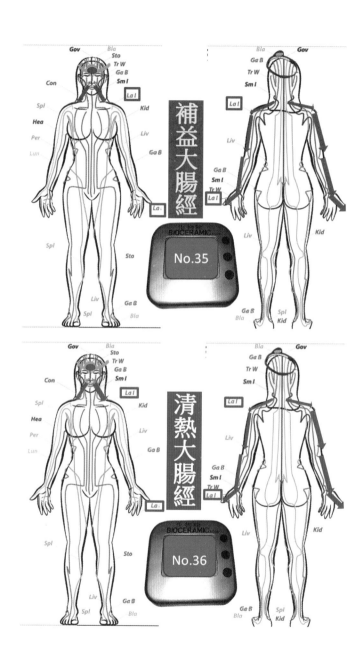

補益大腸經

No.35

清熱大腸經

No.36

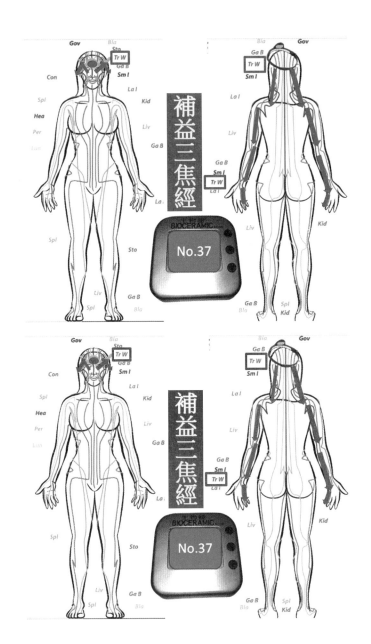

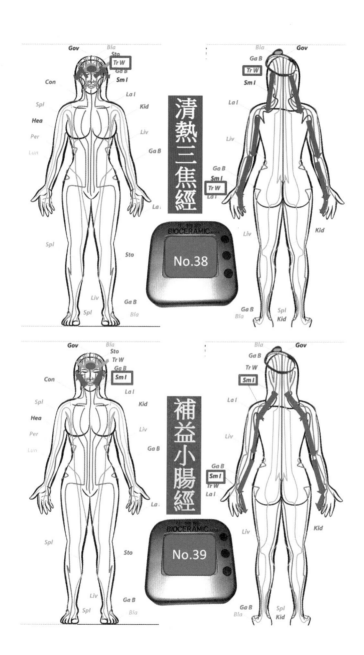

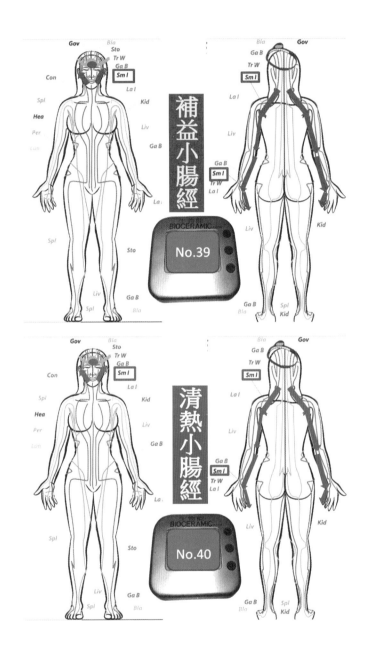

補益小腸經

No.39

清熱小腸經

No.40

213

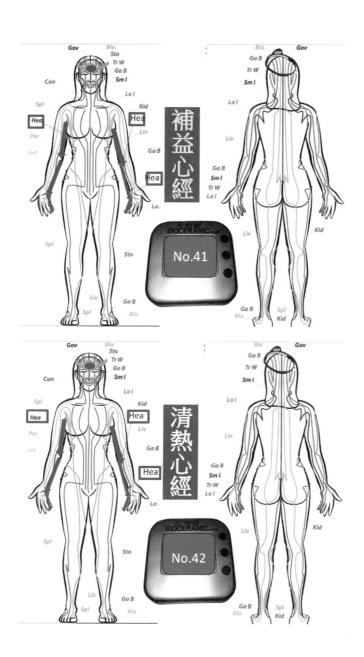

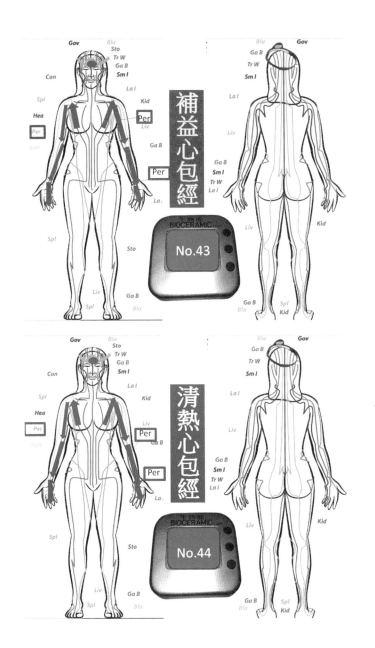

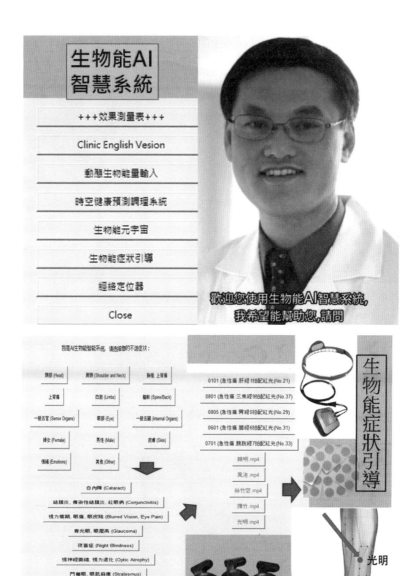

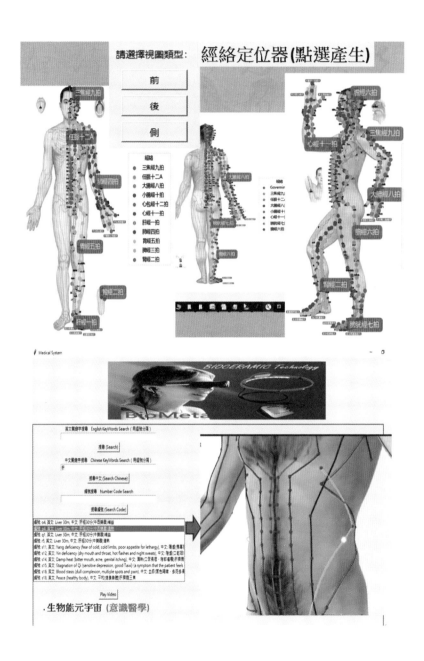

請選擇視圖類型： 經絡定位器(點選產生)

前
後
側

· 生物能元宇宙 (意識醫學)

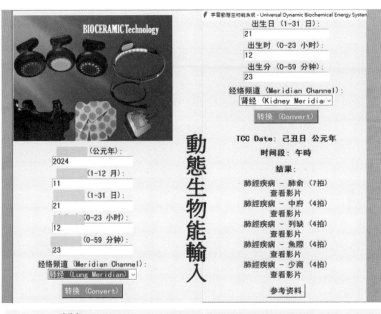

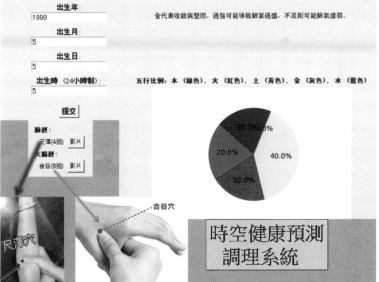

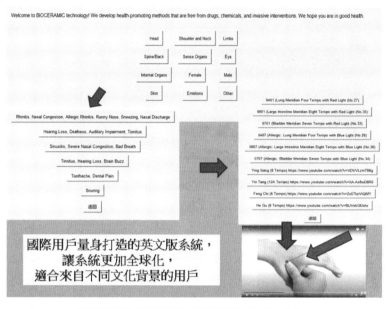

國際用戶量身打造的英文版系統，
讓系統更加全球化，
適合來自不同文化背景的用戶

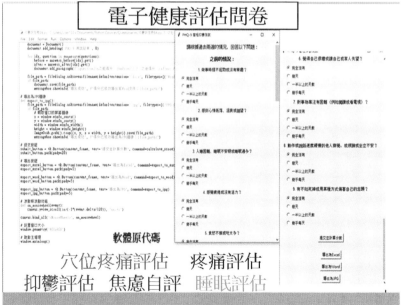

電子健康評估問卷

軟體原代碼

穴位疼痛評估　　疼痛評估
抑鬱評估　　焦慮自評　　睡眠評估

AI機械臂生物光

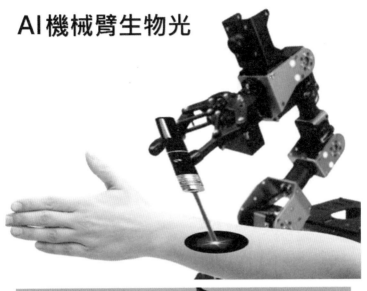

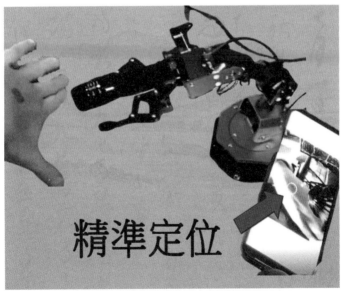

精準定位

執行中與進步中的意識醫學

＜生物能意識腦波＞

隨著科學與醫學的進步，人類對於意識、腦波與醫療應用之間的關聯有了更深入的理解。意識醫學結合了神經科學、生物能分頻腦電波刺激與分析方法，為身心健康和教育提供了嶄新的科學基礎與應用範疇。本文將探討意識醫學的核心原理、科學驗證及實際應用，並闡述其在執行過程中的挑戰與進步。

1.意識與腦波的科學基礎

意識醫學的理論相關於對分頻腦電波的研究。腦波是大腦神經元活動所產生的電流波動，其頻率分為 δ 波 (0.1-4 Hz)、θ 波 (4-8 Hz)、α 波 (8-12 Hz) 和 β 波 (12-30 Hz)。每種類型的腦波與不同的心理、生理狀態相關：

- δ 波：主要出現在深度睡眠狀態，負責身體修復與免疫系統的強化。
- θ 波：與深沉放鬆和潛意識活動相關，有助於記憶的鞏固與學習的啟動。
- α 波：清醒放鬆時占主導地位，有助於思考和學習，是溝通意識與潛意識的橋梁。
- β 波：代表高度的專注與清醒狀態，但過高時可能與壓力和焦慮相關。

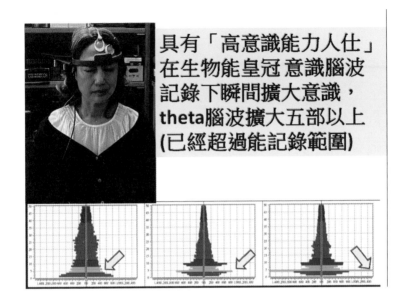

具有「高意識能力人仕」
在生物能皇冠意識腦波
記錄下瞬間擴大意識，
theta腦波擴大五部以上
(已經超過能記錄範圍)

(一)生物能皇冠與松果體的研究與應用

　　松果體被稱為人體的"第三隻眼"，其主要功能是調節褪黑激素的分泌，從而影響睡眠、情緒和生物節律。科學研究表明，通過光線、聲音或腦波的刺激，可以調節松果體的功能，進而影響大腦的意識狀態。

　　本文探討一種名為生物能皇冠的創新裝置。該裝置據稱通過特定的生物能參數刺激松果體，進而調節人體的生理和心理功能。生物能皇冠在運作時會產生特定的振動頻率，這些頻率與人體的腦波以及地球的舒曼共振（Schumann resonance）相互作用，對松果體產生深層的刺激效果。

(二)七色光照射與生物陶瓷能量

此外，生物能皇冠結合了七色光的照射，利用生物陶瓷能量來增強效果。七色光對應紅、橙、黃、綠、藍、靛、紫七種顏色，傳統上與人體的七個能量中心（即脈輪）相關。通過特定波長的彩色光照射，生物能皇冠聲稱能夠與松果體和其他生理系統產生交互作用，進而提升認知表現和心理健康。

目前，關於彩色光照射對松果體和人體生理功能的影響，缺乏充分的科學研究和實驗證據。生物陶瓷能量的概念在科學界也沒有得到廣泛認可，其作用機制需要進一步的研究。

(三)神經化學調控和意識狀態

生物能皇冠的運作機制被聲稱是通過調節松果體內的神經化學過程，以提升其功能。例如，GABA（γ-氨基丁酸）在中樞神經系統中作為主要的抑制性神經遞質，能夠穩定神經系統，減少焦慮情緒。據稱，生物能皇冠的特定振頻可以促進 GABA 的活性，增強其抑制過度神經興奮的效果。此外，該裝置還聲稱能夠優化食欲素（Orexin）的釋放，從而改善使用者的警覺性、清醒狀態和代謝平衡。在刺激松果體的過程中，據稱有助於調節血清素（Serotonin），這可能對情緒穩定、認知能力和生理功能產生影響。

(四)松果體功能的研究與非侵入性生物能技術的應用

松果體是人體中一個小而重要的腺體，位於大腦的中央深處，被認為是調節荷爾蒙分泌和意識狀態的關鍵結構。它能夠利用常用胺基酸之一的色胺酸（Tryptophan）進行一系列生化轉化，生成對人體身心功能至關重要的化學物質，包括血清素（Serotonin）、退黑激素（Melatonin）以及可能存在的 DMT（N,N-二甲基色胺）。這些物質在調節情緒、睡眠、晝夜節律以及精神意識方面發揮著重要作用。本文將探討我們所發展的非侵入性生物能技術，如何透過彩光能量與生物能共振來刺激松果體，提升其對人體的調節能力。

首先，松果體將色胺酸代謝為血清素，這是一種與情緒穩定和幸福感密切相關的神經遞質。血清素的充足水平有助於減少焦慮情緒，增強正面心情，並改善壓力應對能力。然而，現代生活中的壓力和不良生活習慣往往導致血清素水平失衡，進而引發情緒波動與心理健康問題。通過非侵入性的生物陶瓷共振技術，我們可以利用特定的振動頻率來促進松果體內色胺酸代謝途徑的活化，從而提高血清素的生成效率，幫助恢復情緒穩定。

接下來，血清素在松果體中進一步代謝為退黑激素，這是一種調節晝夜節律的荷爾蒙，對於維持健康的睡眠模式和代謝平衡至關重要。退黑激素的分泌受光線強度的影響，在黑暗環境下分泌量增加，幫助人體進入

深度睡眠。我們的彩光能量技術通過模擬自然光線的不同波長，特別是在黃昏和黎明時段的光譜，可以有效地協助松果體適應環境變化，進一步優化退黑激素的分泌節律，從而改善睡眠質量和全身代謝功能。

　　此外，松果體可能參與合成內源性 DMT（N,N-二甲基色胺），這種物質被認為與高層次的精神意識體驗相關，可能在直覺、深層意識甚至幻覺中扮演重要角色。雖然內源性 DMT 的存在與功能仍在科學研究中，但它被認為對意識的非凡狀態具有深遠影響。我們的技術結合彩光與共振模擬，通過與松果體內化學結構的共鳴，可能誘導使用者進入更高層次的意識狀態，而不需依賴任何藥物介入。這種方式既安全又創新，為探索人類意識的潛能提供了一條新途徑。

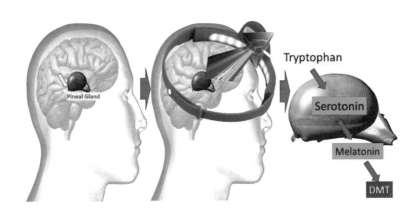

(五)潛在的意識狀態改變

有研究者觀察到，生物能皇冠對某些特定人群可能產生類似於亞馬遜傳統藥物"死藤水"（Ayahuasca）的效應。死藤水以其可能刺激松果體、誘發深層意識狀態的效果而廣為人知。生物能皇冠聲稱通過非侵入式的方法達到類似的目的，其振頻設計據稱與松果體內可能存在的內源性 DMT（N,N-二甲基色胺）產生共振，誘導使用者進入更高層次的意識狀態。然而，內源性 DMT 在人體中的作用仍是一個有爭議且尚未完全了解的領域，需要更多的科學研究來加以證實。

總之，生物能皇冠據稱通過不同的生物陶瓷共振與經絡系統產生共鳴，以及利用七色光的照射，結合生物陶瓷能量，與松果體和其他生理系統形成直接聯繫。這些聲稱的功能包括神經化學調控、意識狀態的誘導和生理功能的提升。目前，雖有多篇研究論文從實證醫學的角度探討其效果，但仍需更多的科學研究和臨床試驗來驗證其有效性和安全性。

2 生物能皇冠與聲光腦波刺激技術

為了實現意識醫學的應用，科學家開發了結合聲光音的腦波調節設備，例如生物能皇冠。這是一種能發射特定光頻與聲音模式的裝置，旨在刺激腦波以達到平衡和修復的效果。在治療中，患者佩戴生物能皇冠，通過預設的光頻（如綠光、紅光）與聲音節拍，協助調節異

常的腦波頻率。例如，使用 α 波誘導放鬆，或透過降低 β 波水平來減少壓力。

臨床實驗表明，此方法在改善睡眠、減輕焦慮以及提升學習能力方面具有顯著成效。例如，針對注意力缺失與多動症（ADHD）的兒童，腦波調節技術能降低過高的 β 波，幫助患者恢復專注力。此外，對於慢性失眠的患者，通過引導 δ 波進入深度睡眠，也展現了良好的臨床效果。

3.科學驗證與應用成效

意識醫學的一個重要特徵是其客觀的科學驗證。研究中常使用分頻率腦電波圖（qEEG）來記錄治療前後的腦波變化，進行量化分析。例如，特定生物能光頻調理後，患者的 α 波顯著增強，伴隨著放鬆程度的提高。另一項實驗表明，透過聲光治療，91.7% 的實驗組患者出現 β 波的顯著降低，顯示其壓力指數明顯下降。在教育和特殊需求的應用中，意識醫學提供了一種創新的干預方法。例如，在自閉症譜系障礙和學習障礙的干預中，腦波調節技術幫助患者改善情緒波動，增強記憶力與學習能力。這些成效不僅來自患者的主觀回饋，也通過腦波數據得以驗證。

4.執行與挑戰-----未來展望

儘管意識醫學在科學基礎和臨床應用上均展現出巨大潛力，其執行過程仍面臨多項挑戰。首先，如何確保

設備的安全性與標準化，是未來推廣的關鍵。其次，不同患者的腦波特性和反應差異，要求治療方案更具個性化。此外，對於遠端治療的需求，如何結合人工智能與數據分析技術，實現即時監控與個性化調節，仍是目前亟待解決的問題。

展望未來，意識醫學有望結合神經網絡建模與大數據技術，提供更精準的意識狀態調控。此外，在醫療與教育領域的跨界合作，將促進其在心理健康、學習輔助與腦疾病治療中的廣泛應用。

5.結論

意識醫學作為一門結合科學與醫療的前沿學科，正在重新定義人類對意識、腦波與健康之間關係的認識。通過生物能皇冠和腦波調節技術，其不僅在科學驗證中表現出色，更在教育與醫療實踐中展現了廣闊的應用前景。隨著科技的進步，意識醫學將進一步推動人類對自我意識與健康潛力的探索與發展。

生物能遠距意識干預

艾德加·米切爾（Edgar Mitchell）是美國 1971 年阿波羅 14 號的宇航員，也是第六位登上月球表面的人。他在太空飛船上進行了一系列未經 NASA 批准的私人超感知實驗（ESP），探索人類意識與宇宙間的潛在連結。返回地球後，他在加利福尼亞州北部創立了心

靈科學研究所（Noetic Institute of Sciences），致力於研究人類意識的深層潛力及其對科學和靈性發展的意義。

遠距意識干預的理論與實踐

遠距意識干預是一項以意識能量為基礎的科學探索，旨在證明人類意識不受時空限制，具有跨地域的影響力。透過遠距實驗，干預者和被干預者同時佩戴生物能皇冠，並根據預設參數進行調控，觀察干預是否能誘發對方的心理與生理反應。這些實驗的核心是驗證人類意識能否通過特定的能量場進行非接觸式的互動和影響。

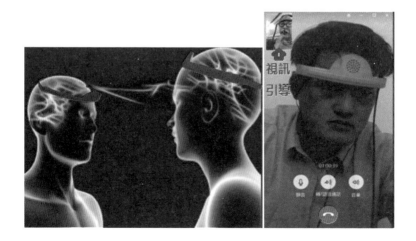

高意識人力的重要角色

在干預過程中，具有「高意識能力人仕」干預者起到了關鍵作用。他們能夠以更強的專注力與能量感知能力，幫助對方進入特定的意識狀態，誘導情緒變化及身體上的心理和生理反應。例如，干預者可以引導被干預者感到平靜、喜悅，甚至促進身體的放鬆與恢復。

實驗與觀察的進展

我們已經完成多次相關的實驗觀察，結果顯示遠距干預能在一定程度上影響被干預者的狀態。這些實驗中，干預者通過手機或其他通訊軟體 APP 進行遠程操作，突破了國界和地理限制，實現了真正的無邊界干預。

新方向與未來展望

生物能遠距意識干預的研究為醫療、心理健康和意識提升領域帶來了嶄新的可能性。未來的研究可以進一步量化干預效果，探索更精準的干預參數，以及對意識連結的持續性和深度影響進行分析。此外，如何將這一技術應用於特殊教育、壓力管理及疾病康復，將是下一步的重要發展方向。

透過這一創新技術，我們不僅看到了意識的廣闊潛

能，更重塑了人類對自身與宇宙連結的認知。這是一項跨越科學與靈性界限的研究，為未來人類意識的發展鋪平了道路。

遠端意識實例

一位小學特教女老師遇到二年級班上一位過動症男同學，小 J 同學。他在課堂中經常表現出暴力破壞行為，曾接受教育局和社會局的介入調查，最終被認定具有反社會人格。小 J 同學從小父母離異，父親長期不在家，由祖父母照顧成長。

經介紹，小 J 同學加入生物能意識實驗研究。研究方式採用配戴生物能皇冠，參與者包括小 J 同學本人、特教美雲老師和一位高意識的管老師。三位參與者分別位於台灣桃園市與上海市。

實驗中，參與者首先將生物能皇冠設定為「紫光膽經六拍」參數。該參數可與人體 α 腦波（8-12 Hz）以及地表和電離層間的全球性電磁頻譜舒曼波（Schumann resonance，約 8-10 Hz）產生共振，進一步促進可能存在的意識能量傳遞。

三位主要參與者同時啟動相同的參數，位於上海市的管老師開始感應到訊息，並提出問題：「小 J 同學，你晚上為什麼會常常起來？」小 J 同學未能理解其含義，但他的祖母明白，並協助回答：「他晚上會夢遊，

常常不由自主地起來。」接著，管老師提出另一個問題：

「小 J 同學，針對你對班上的那位小朋友，是否可以不要對他生氣？」當時，在場的其他人未能理解管老師的意思，但小 J 同學突然激動起來，大聲說道：

「不行！不行！我無法原諒他！」經深入了解後，得知小 J 同學班上有一位亞斯伯格症的小孩。由於該小孩為輕度自閉症，他特別喜歡接近小 J 同學，並經常表現出友善親近的舉動。然而，小 J 同學對這些行為非常反感，甚至極度討厭該小孩。首次實驗基本上成功找出了問題的關鍵。接下來的三週內，每週進行兩次相同的實驗，但改由台灣方面主導。由於疫情期間無法直接面對面交流，實驗均以視訊方式進行，並由三地分開同步執行。實驗的核心是透過美云老師、高意識管老師以及醫生，與病人本身進行遠端意識交流，以減少他對同學之間的誤會，並緩解不當的情緒投射。此外，實驗還進行了腦波測試，結果顯示小 J 同學對班上那位同學的怨恨已完全消失，且對其行為不再在意。同時，意識腦波實驗也取得了良好的進展，顯示出顯著的改善效果。

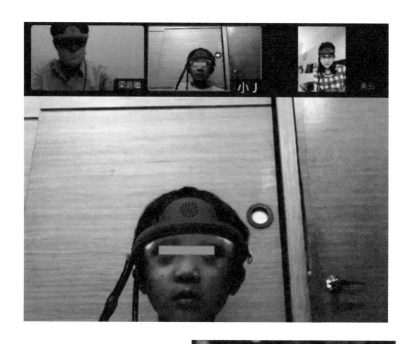

生物能皇冠使用前後之分頻率意識:明顯α波、δ波及θ波增加,代表專心度增加和動度下降

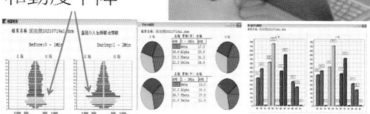

集體潛意識真實存在與實驗記錄

這是關於 T 小姐的介紹，以及一次有關生物能意識擴張的實驗過程。T 小姐在童年時曾經歷過一個特殊的情境，當時她感受到某種不測的預兆，看到了她的哥哥身上發生了一些異常情況。結果，她的哥哥遭受了一次重大意外，幸運的是他最終平安存活，並在幾年後逐漸康復。這段經歷讓 T 小姐對生命與人生有了許多深入的思考。與她相識後，我發現她具有特別的氣質與靈性特徵，於是讓她嘗試使用皇冠裝置進行刺激，並結合冥想的引導。在短短的實驗中，她描述看到許多圖形與符號，並感覺自己進入了一個全新的空間。因此，我進一步邀請她參與共振實驗。在實驗過程中，她提到看到一串古文字，並將其形容為咒語。

雖然 T 小姐是基督徒，但她對舊約聖經並不熟悉，對古猶太文化的了解也非常有限。在了解這些情況後，有一天我突發奇想，讓她觀看了一些我學習過的希伯來文字。沒想到，她在看到這些文字時，不僅再次聯想到咒語，還表示感受到了一種祝福的能量，這似乎在指引她一條正確的道路。

然而，對 T 小姐來說，她始終覺得生活中缺乏清晰的方向。她認為這些訊息可能並非針對她個人，而是與設計這項共振實驗的人或背後的意志有關，也許這與

我有關。不過，對於這些假設，我並未特別介意，甚至也無法證實這種可能性。為了更進一步驗證，我安排了一次規模更大的共振刺激實驗，然而這需要使用醫院內非常昂貴且繁忙的設備。經過多方協調後，終於找到時間完成實驗。實驗安排前一日，我想到是否能在實驗後，讓她觀看一段虛擬情境的影片來進一步檢驗她的回憶。為此，我花時間製作了一段影片，其中包含希伯來文字、古代與現代以色列的文化風情，以及民謠音樂。

在實驗當天，過程分為兩部分。根據 T 小姐的描述，開始時，她感到被一股強大的力量拉到了一個遙遠的空間，看到地球從遠處的景象。隨後，她又看到了一座金黃色的建築物。實驗結束後，我安排她觀看預先準備的影片，結果驚人地發現，她所描述的金黃色建築正是影片中耶路撒冷第三聖殿的 3D 設計圖。實驗完成後，T 小姐的狀況穩定，但在第三天的夢境中，她描述看見了一個黑色的盒子，上面刻有雕紋，並伴隨著搶奪盒子的激烈情節。在夢中，她聽到兩次聲音，似乎暗示這個盒子真實存在。這被認為是舊約聖經中提到的「約櫃」，與摩西的故事密切相關，但其下落早已成為未解之謎。

總結而言，次實驗的過程與以往有所不同。過去我通常是觀察特殊人群的擴張現象，但這次我深刻地感受到自身與這種現象之間的互動與聯繫。這一切令人深

思，或許生物能意識擴張不僅僅是一種個體經驗，更可能牽涉到集體潛意識的層面。在我們以研究報告的形式發表的論文中，其中一個研究室針對生物共振與意識擴張（ESP）的現象進行了深入探討。此研究特別引用了佛洛伊德的學生著名心理學和精神醫學科學專家：卡爾·榮格（Carl Jung）關於集體潛意識的相關理論作為基礎。而我們的研究方向則聚焦於醫學工程及儀器設備所產生的物理性刺激，這是一種目前較為獨特的探索方式，為意識擴張研究提供了全新的視角。

十二銅人經絡代表穴位

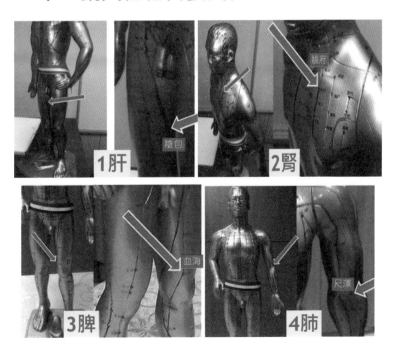

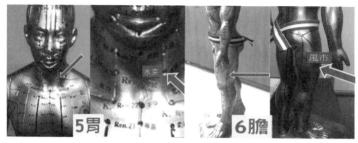

5胃　水突　Ren 22 天突　Ren 21 璇璣　6膽　風市

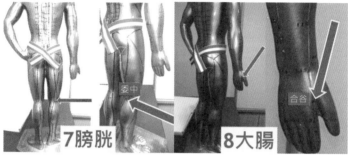

7膀胱　委中　8大腸　合谷

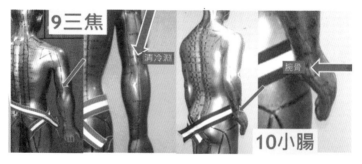

9三焦　清冷淵　腕骨　10小腸

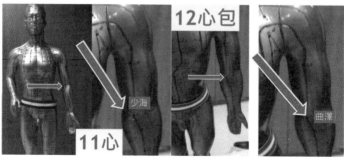

12心包　11心　少海　曲澤

<網站 QR Code>

生物能 e 學院網站 QR Code

生物能軟體系統(光能貼片/元宇宙) QR Code

AI 生物能 FB QRcode

AI 生物能客服 QRcode

AI 生物能課程 QRcode

生物能商城 QRcode

國家圖書館出版品預行編目(CIP)資料

意識醫學生物能 AI = Introduction the technology of consciousness medicine/ 梁庭繼作 . -- 一版 . -- 臺北市 ： 健康管理顧問有限公司 , 2024.12
　面 ； 　公分
ISBN 978-986-87120-6-5(平裝)

1.CST：生物醫學 2.CST：醫療科技 3.CST：中西醫整合

410.1636　　　　　　　　　　113019982

意識醫學 生物能AI

作者:梁庭繼　醫師
發行所:健康管理顧問有限公司
出版者:健康管理顧問有限公司
電話:(02)2357-0889
傳真:(02)2357-0905
E-mail:health2475@gmail.com
地址:台北市杭州南路一段115號7樓之5
出版:一版一刷 2024.12　　　　訂價:500元

本系統並非提供醫學診斷和治療所使用